AF540755

COMMUNICATION STRATEGIES IN REPRODUCTIVE HEALTH
(AN IMPACT ANALYSIS IN A TRIBAL COMMUNITY)

COMMUNICATION STRATEGIES IN REPRODUCTIVE HEALTH

(AN IMPACT ANALYSIS IN A TRIBAL COMMUNITY)

By

Dr. Benazir Patil

Ph.D.

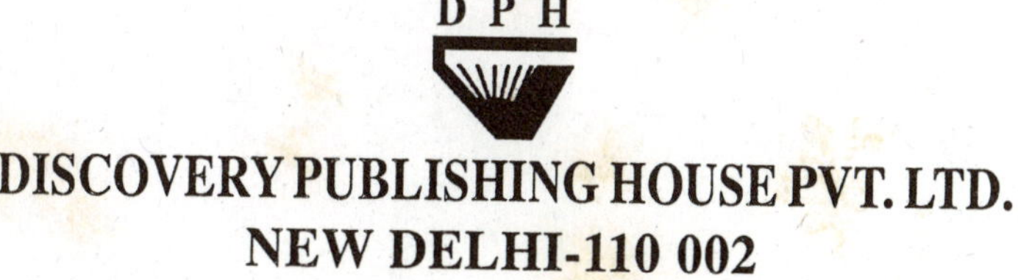

DISCOVERY PUBLISHING HOUSE PVT. LTD.

NEW DELHI-110 002

First Published-2009

ISBN 978-81-8356-379-6

Published by

DISCOVERY PUBLISHING HOUSE PVT. LTD.
4831/24, Ansari Road, Prahlad Street
Darya Ganj, New Delhi-110002 (India)
Phone: 23279245 • Fax: 91-11-23253475
E-mail: dphbooks@rediffmail.com
dphtemp@indiatimes.com
website: www.discoverypublishing.com

Printed at:

Sachin Printers
Delhi

Dedicated
To
My Beloved Mother

Preface

After a complete decade of work in the post International Conference on Population and Development (ICPD) scenario, several governments have sought opportunities and have reviewed the progress towards the conference's 20-year goals. The Cairo program enlarged the scope of earlier population policies and called on governments to look at family planning services in the context of comprehensive reproductive health care. The ICPD identified advocacy and information, education and communication (IEC) as important elements for raising awareness on population and reproductive health (including sexual health and family planning) issues and in mobilizing government and public support for the achievement of the goals and objectives of the ICPD Programme of Action (POA).

In India the clearest impact of the ICPD has been its elimination of method-specific targets, an action taken in April 1996. Now India is committed to several new initiatives, components of these initiatives were incorporated into the 1997 Reproductive and Child Health Project, which, with World Bank collaboration, was initiating a district-based planning approach to create an integrated health delivery system. In India too IEC strategies are being applied in communicating with women so that they are able to have control of their bodies (e.g. control over the risk of STDs, able to negotiate with men to use condoms to avoid pregnancy, prevent the risk of STD/ HIV.) and are able to understand the changes within themselves and their bodies as they pass through various phases of the reproductive cycle.

Communication, specifically in health is a **process** for partnership and participation that is based on two-way dialogue, where there is an interactive interchange of information, ideas, techniques and knowledge between senders and receivers of information on an equal footing, leading to improved understanding, shared knowledge, greater consensus, and identification of possible effective action. This publication attempts to analyze the impact of several such communication strategies that were applied for extension, awareness and information sharing with the tribal women of Melghat region, especially after the 1993 infant mortality crisis and as per the comprehensive RCH program in the state of Maharashtra.

The book comprises of chapters that focus on: Theoretical Framework of public health policy; History and Evolution of Health Policies; Communication Strategies in Reproductive Health; Administrative structures and Information Education and Communication Programs in Melghat Region; about NGOs in Health communication; Implementation mechanisms of health policy; Public Health Care Programs in the state of Maharashtra; Communication Strategies used in a tribal community in Melghat region; Impact Analysis; and Conclusions and recommendations.

Acknowledgements

Authoring this book has been a wonderful and rewarding experience. However, it would not have been possible without the help and guidance of a few important people.

I owe the most to my beloved mother, who is not here with me today. She has always been a source of inspiration to me especially with regard to academic expertise. Without her immense persuasion, I would not have been where I am!

While conducting the research, I have received inspiration, encouragement, help and support from many people. I record my deep gratitude to all of them. I would have wished to give full and fair recognition to all of the people from whom I derived help, but that has practical difficulties, which force me to be content without mentioning their names.

I have received immense help, guidance and inspiration from my teachers Dr. (Mrs.) Nalini Paranjape and Prof. Shrikant Paranjape. Without their initiation and constant supervision, it would not have been possible to complete my work. It was their personal commitment to my work that remained a continuing source of inspiration to me to complete this study.

I am also indebted to all the government officials at all levels working for the Maharashtra State Public Health Department, without their permission and support, this research could not have been brought to fruition. Special thanks are extended to Dr. Subhash Salunkhe, the Director General of Health Services, Maharashtra, Mr. Naveen Kumar, Principal Secretary, Public Health, Government of Maharashtra, Dr. Manmohan Singh, Principal Secretary – Family

Welfare, Government of Maharashtra, and Mr. Digvijay Khanvilkar, Health Minister, Maharashtra State.

I extend thanks to Ms. Veena Panse in assisting me for statistical analysis.

I thank all the couples from the Melghat villages and the employees of the PHC, Semadoh, who cooperated with me and answered the cumbersome questionnaires.

My constant source of inspiration, my father, mother, brother, mother-in-law and father-in-law showed great care and concern for the timely completion of my work.

I cannot complete this acknowledgement without mentioning the name of my husband, Deepak, who always supported me and stood by me thereby making this period smooth sailing. To my son, Roshan, I owe a loving apology for not being able to keep up with the demands that an eight year old would place on his mother.

Benazir Patil

Contents

1

Introduction

Scope of the Book

This book looks at the Public Health Policy of Government of India since its independence with a specific focus on the communication strategies used to implement the policies. Since, there has been no separate Reproductive Health Policy in India, the focus is on different policy documents and the conclusions related to efforts in Reproductive Health have been derived accordingly. The policy documents viz. National Family Planning Program of 1951-52; Different committees and commissions for health reforms; National Health policy – 1983; National Population Policy – 2000; and Health related planning in each five-year plan have been studied.

Within the purview of Public Health Policy the study focuses on the following:

- Policy evolution in India with regards to Public Health.
- Policy formulation and implementation processes in the field of Public Health.
- The emphasis laid down on the policies related to Reproductive Health in particular.
- The evolution of the Health Education programs in India, the communication campaigns undertaken and the strategies applied in the field of Reproductive Health.

- The policy implementation with regards to Reproductive Health done in the Melghat region of Maharashtra as a case study.
- The impact analyses of the Health Education efforts and communication strategies applied in the Melghat region.

The Selection of the Area for the Study of the Implementation Process is Based on the Several Reasons

- The issue related to malnutrition in the Melghat region in 1993 compelled the state and the central government to pay more attention to child health in the area. This automatically triggered the concentration on maternal health in the region and accordingly led to the emergence of a number of schemes and policy statements.
- The schemes focused upon health inputs, information and care of the pregnant mothers, nursing mothers and the women in general – the prospective mothers in reproductive age.

All the schemes and programs implemented in last one decade have been studied here and the impact these schemes have made on the lives of the women in reproductive age has been analyzed.

The findings of the impact analysis list out the following:

1. Information and awareness that the couples from reproductive age possess regarding their general health.
2. Specific information that the couples from reproductive age have acquired regarding Reproductive Health.
3. The changes occurred amongst the tribal population in attitudes and practices due to the Information, Education and Communication programs.
4. The benefits derived by the women through the schemes.
5. The impediments and hassles the communicators (health functionaries – implementers) face in implementation of the policies.
6. The opinions and views of the policy makers.

I. The Rationale for this Research Study

The present study is an attempt to study the Public Health policies of the government of India and analyze the impact of communication strategies applied in the field of Reproductive Health. The formulation of Public Health policies in our country has been a result of recommendations of the reports submitted by different committees from time to time. The Public Health policies of independent India since 1947 are a British legacy predominantly based on the report submitted by the Health Survey and Development Committee under the chairmanship of Sir Joseph Bhore in the year 1946. Almost all the committees, missions and study groups focused on the pressing issues of population explosion and the severe mortality and morbidity of children and women. The focus on the area of Maternal and Child Health was actually a process to confront these two issues. Specifically the National Family Planning Program of 1952, National Health Policy 1983 and the National Population Policy 2000, have focused on the Reproductive Health of women extensively. However, the changing scenarios of world conferences and international efforts in the area of maternal health have resulted in it being referred to as Reproductive Health, the actual watershed coming in the year 1994 at the time of the International Conference on Population and Development.

As early as 1952, when the first Public Health Program (the National Family Planning Program) was launched, Health Education was identified as the most necessary and critical tool to implement the enacted policies. The importance of it and the various strategies of information and communication were suggested in each Five Year Plan. With the changing trends and the changing national and international scenarios, each of the policy has had new arenas to be focused and new strategies to be applied. Similarly, there has been a change in the population policy from targets and quotas to a broader Reproductive Health agenda, encouraging choice and quality care.

It is important and necessary to point out the gaps between our policy and implementation processes to the policy makers, specifically with regard to the application of communication strategies in the field of Reproductive Health, so that the problems of voiceless women from the remote parts of our country belonging to the most vulnerable sections of the society reach the policy makers and result in raising the efficiency of implementation through these inputs. Developing countries like India need information bases created through independent, objective research as an input for effective policy making and for implementation of programs to improve the Reproductive Health of its population.

The findings of the research project shall help study the impact of the communication strategies applied and programs implemented as a part of the policy of the government in the field of Reproductive Health (falling into the category of Health and Family Welfare). It will also help understand the behaviour changes, attitudes, understanding and responses of the people to the strategies applied and programs implemented.

II. Objectives of the Study

It is important to study the implementation process of these enacted policies. Against the background of the comprehensive policies, the present research study intends to analyze the implementation of these policies through impact assessment of communication strategies being applied in the field of Reproductive Health. These questions would be addressed in the broader perspective of the social, political and economic environment in which the policy process is rooted.

The basic objectives of the research on impact assessment of the various communication strategies and programs related to Reproductive Health in Maharashtra are as follows:

- To analyze the policies of the government on the basis of communication methods and strategies for the effective implementation of Reproductive Health Programs.
- To study the impact of the communication strategies applied as a part of policy of the government.
- To study the problems and gaps related to the effects of implementation of Information Education and Communication (IEC) strategies.
- To study the mindset of the communicator and the problems faced by him or her in communicating to the people.

- To understand the present IEC techniques of the Reproductive and Child Health program and other related programs of the govt. of India.

III. Research Methodology

The **basic assumptions** of the study on impact analysis of the various communication strategies applied and the various schemes extended in the field of Reproductive Health are stated in the research design. These relate to:

1. Why the various communication strategies applied in the field of Reproductive Health in Maharashtra have succeeded or failed?
2. Why are the various schemes introduced for the couple falling in the reproductive age in Maharashtra have succeeded or failed?
3. What are the causal socio-cultural, administrative, managerial and financial factors for the success or failure of the strategies and the schemes?
4. Whether the strategies applied and schemes implemented in Maharashtra have some inherent weakness and do these require any modification suitable to socio cultural peculiarities of the region?
5. Goes into the related questions like inadequacy of implementation, administrative failure in reaching the benefits, lack of convergence of the schemes etc.

Universe

The location of the study is Chikhaldara block of Amravati district of Maharashtra state. Chikhaldara block is completely tribal in nature and the data has been collected from fifteen villages of this block. Chikhaldara is a part of the Melghat forest area of Amravati, about 100 km from the district head quarters and is a remote tribal belt consisting of tribes called Korkus and Gonds. Both are Hindi speaking tribes with low level of literacy, mal-nourished, and cut off from the main stream.

Sampling Frame and Procedure

In Maharashtra, Amravati is a tribal district with the total area of 12,210 sq. kms. and tribal population of 316,448 as per the 1991 census[1]. In the field of health it is chosen for the purpose of study for two reasons, it has one of the largest population of tribal, and is known for its malnutrition problem, which had cropped up in the nineties. The sampling was done randomly as per the grid pattern as far as the people from the villages were concerned.

Sample Size

From each village about 10–15 couples were interviewed making it to about 200 couples (400 people) from 15 villages of Amravati district. The officials from the district level DHO office, block level PHC were interviewed. Panchayati Raj representatives, educated villagers, social workers, NGO workers, anganwadi workers constitute the units of observations.

The data collected from the structured questionnaires was supplemented with the news reports related to public health published in the local newspapers. Further, information was collected from the offices of the State Family Welfare Bureau, Pune; Directorate of Health Services, Mumbai and Pune; Mantralaya, Mumbai; State Information, Education and Communication Bureau, Pune, District IEC unit and Melghat cell, Amravati; Zilla Parishad – Amravati, District Health Office – Amravati, Panchayat Samiti Office – Chikhaldara, PHC Office-Semadoh, Chikhaldara; and the ITDP Office – Dharni, Amravati. The Five Year Plan documents and the performance budget documents were taken from the Yashwantrao Chavan Development Academy, Pune. Formal discussions were held with the State Health Minister – Maharashtra, Principal Secretary-Public Health – Maharashtra, Principal Secretary-Family Welfare – Maharashtra, Director General of Health Services, Assistant Director, Directorate of Health Services, Mumbai, and the Additional Director, Assistant Director – State Family Welfare Bureau, Pune.

Tools for Data Collection

Three separate interview schedules were prepared in English – one each for couples, officials, and the Secretarial/Ministerial candidates. The interview schedules comprised of mostly structured, close ended and a few open-ended questions. The schedules were pre-tested and standardized.

Data Collection and Analysis

All the interview schedules have been coded and a separate codebook has been prepared for each. The data has been checked for the gaps, organized and coded with the help of a codebook. Codes have been assigned to various responses, which have been categorized and similar responses have been collapsed and coded as one. Data has been coded on the computer code sheet, then fed into the computer and processed for statistical analysis through the use of SPSS software package. In order to study the objectives listed a tabulation plan has been evolved following which the data has been analyzed on the computer.

Extensive informal discussions were held with the District Health Officer and the officials from DHO office and the PHC so as to gain the insights into the problems of the implementation of various policy level decisions. Discussions were held with the Deputy Chief Executive Officer, Amravati, and the NGOs working in the field of health.

Local newspapers were scanned for news about policy statements or issues in Public Health. Government Reports on the performance budget; Five Year Plan documents of Government of India; National Health Policy – 1983; National Population policy – 2000; State Plans of Government of Maharashtra; Program of Action – International Conference on Population and Development, 1994; reports of the Indian delegations to World Health Assemblies; Annual Reports of Public Health Commissioner in British India; Annual Reports of Ministry of Health and Family Welfare – Government of India; Data of the National Family Health Survey, Maharashtra – 1998-99; Reports on National and International Policy Projects in different states of India; articles from various journals; Health status – Maharashtra – 2002-2003; RCH program (guidelines) – Schemes for implementation – 1997; Manual on Community Needs Assessment Approach in Family Welfare Program – MOHFW – GOI; Planning Commission documents; Report of the WHO commission on health and environment – WHO – 1992; and the reports of the national and international conferences held in last 20 years with regards to Public Health and other publications were referred to as secondary data.

General health practices, information and awareness regarding Reproductive Health, Reproductive Health problems faced by men and women, sources and types of information and communication, impact occurring due to the received information and education were some of the aspects on which information was collected through primary data.

IV. Selection of the Area

Brief History of the District

Amravati, originally a part of the Berar Province in British India became a part of Madhya Pradesh in the independent India. The district was transferred from Madhya Pradesh to Bombay State during the reorganization of states in the year 1956. The district forms a part of Maharashtra state since 1st May 1960.

The total area of Amravati district is 12,210 sq.km. and the total population of 2,200,257. Amravati district has 1996 villages out of which 1681 villages are inhabited and 315 villages are uninhabited. Chikhaldara is the largest block in terms of number of villages and geographical area accounting for 10.05 per cent of the total inhabited villages and 4.93 per cent of the total rural population of the district. Within the thirteen blocks of the district, per centage of the small sized (less than 500) villages is the highest in Chikhaldara block.

The scheduled tribe population in Amravati district comprises of 316,448. The five major tribes in the district are Korku, Gond, Rajgond, Dhanwar, Pardhi and Mahadeo Koli. The literacy rate amongst the scheduled tribes is 44.57% as against the general literacy of 70.06% of the district, however the literacy rate of Chikhaldara block is as low as 27.20%. The sex ratio of the schedule tribes in the district is 947 as against 936 the general sex ratio of the district.

Korku tribe with 141,615 persons is the predominant tribe in the district (44.75%). It is strongly represented in the Dharni and Chikhaldara blocks (89.27%). In language and general type they are said to be identical with the Kols and Santhals. They are divided into many classes viz. Mavasi or Bhowavaya, Bavaria, Ruma and Bondoyas. They are mainly found in the rural areas of the district (98.92%). They mainly speak Korku language. Korku Language belongs to the *Munda* stock of aboriginal language. The phonetical system of Korku is broadly the same as in Santhali. Korkus are the worshippers of the dead and hence outside the village one may find a hut with some painted logs thrust in the ground, these are their gods.

Amravati is administratively divided into 14 blocks out of which Chikhaldara, Achalpur, Anjangaon & Chandurbazar are the blocks having maximum population of adiwasis (Tribal population). As per the epic Mahabharata, Amravati (Indrapuri) is the place from where Rukmini was kidnapped by lord Krishna. Amravati also hails its fame due to the works of social reformers like Sant Gadge Baba, Sant Gulabrao Maharaj & Sant Tukadoji Maharaj and is the land of freedom fighters and social workers like Taraben, Vir Vamanrao Joshi-Dadasaheb Khaparde, Dr. Dajishaheb Patwardhan, Shri. Nanashaheb Gokhale and educational revolutionaries like Dr. Punjabrao Deshmukh. Geographically, the district is divided into two parts, plains around Purna River and the ranges of Satpuda.

Selection of Chikhaldara Block

From the selected Amravati district, the Chikhaldara block was selected for intensive study as this block is considered to be one of the most densely populated tribal areas of the district. Chikhaldara is 100 kilometers away from the district by road. The block consists of tribal population 57,798, which consists of Korkus and Gonds. The percentage of scheduled tribe population in the district is 18.26 per cent. This is mainly concentrated in Chikhaldara block.

Chikhaldara being hill station and rich in nature, beauty and wild life is a famous tourist center since the declaration of Melghat Tiger Project by the Government of India. The tribal people like Korkus, Gonds and Gavalis still maintain a traditional life here and appear to be far away from the modem civilization. Rainfall varies from 800 mm to 1200 mm in this area. Rice, Pulses and Soya-bean are main Agricultural products. People here are also busy in collecting herbs like Tendupatta-Hirda, Sal, Moha and Bamboo. Many villages are not even connected by road. The area still remains backward due to superstitions. Plains in this area produce Cotton,

Jowar, Soya-bean, oranges etc. but people are completely dependent on rainfall. Chikhaldara, has 53 Gram-panchayats, with 169 (As per 1991 census) villages with 85% non- educated population of the tribals. They meet both ends with the help of agriculture in non-irrigated land, sale of herbs and liquor made out of Moha flowers. The total population of this block is 73,949.

Thus the location of the village or town, proximity to the urban and rural centers, caste composition, settlement patterns, levels of social and economic development, attitude of villagers towards health services, the proximity of the people to the health facilities are some of the important factors which have a close impact on the Reproductive Health of women in the area. Amravati district occupies an important place in the available health infrastructure, implementation of schemes for the tribal areas.

For the district as a whole, the health infrastructure is as follows[2]:

Primary Health Centers	:	56
Primary Health Squads	:	13
Mobile Health Squads	:	8
Sub-Centres	:	320
Ayurvedic Clinics	:	65
Rural Hospitals	:	18

For the District as a Whole, the Health Status is as Follows.

Birthrate	25.07
Death rate	7.42
Infant mortality rate	38.22
Maternal mortality rate	0.45
Couple protection rate	63.15
Sex ratio	975
Registration of pregnant mothers	86%
Non institutional deliveries	61.50%
Institutional deliveries	38.50%
Deliveries conducted by untrained personnel	9%
Deliveries conducted by trained personnel	91%

From the Chikhaldara block, fifteen villages were selected for administering the interview schedules. The criteria for the selection of fifteen villages have mainly been the representative character of the population. Since the government is emphasizing on inputs and health extension in the remote and hilly areas, there are special recommendations and special schemes for the tribal areas, the scheduled tribes and the under privileged. It was imperative that the sample includes this section of the society for the impact of the assessment of the implementation of public health policies related to Reproductive Health. The general population is aware regarding the availability of health services, as well as some of the schemes being extended by the Department of Health and Family Welfare. Some of the Non Governmental Organizations working in the tribal tract have helped in creating awareness amongst the people[3]. The tribals from this tract are covered under the Integrated Tribal Development Project, with the headquarters at Dharni.

District Structure

For administrative purposes at the district level, the Zilla Parishad (ZP) of Amravati district was established on May 1, 1962 as per the three-tier structure of Panchayati Raj. The administration at the block level is managed by 14 Panchayat Samitees in 14 blocks of Amravati, under the purview of ZP. Out of the 14 Panchayat Samitees Chikhaldara and Dharni blocks of Melghat region fall under the purview of Tribal Sub Plan. At the village level the district has 842 Gram Panchayats in 1848 villages. Both the ZP and PS run as per the rules laid down in the Maharashtra ZP and PS Act1961, whereas the Gram Panchayat runs as per the rules laid down in the Mumbai Gram Panchayat Act of 1958.

The Zilla Parishad has 11 committees with different portfolios; health being one of the portfolio. Earlier the ZP did not have a committee on Women and Child development however this has been created after the crisis of infant mortality in the year 1993. ZP comprises of totally 59 elected Zilla Parishad members. The Chief Executive Officer is the administrative head of the district and guides 16 subordinates who function as the heads of the different departments. The 16 officials are; Deputy Chief Executive Officer – General purposes; Deputy Chief Executive Officer – Panchayat; Deputy Chief Executive Officer – Child Welfare – looking after

Integrated Child Development Services (Purak Ahar Yojana). This is the new portfolio created after the infant mortality crisis in 1993; Project Director – District Rural Development Agency – looks after schemes and developmental programs; Executive Engineer – Civil works; Executive Engineer – Irrigation; Executive Engineer – Water Supply; District Health Officer; District Animal Husbandry Officer; District Social Welfare Officer; Chief Accounts and Finance Officer; Extension Officer - Primary; Extension Officer - Secondary; Extension Officer – Adult Education; Age Development Officer; and Women and Child Development Officer.

Inspection Machinery in Health at the District Level

The inspection machinery in health within the district has several wings. Firstly, the District Health Officer leads the inspection machinery in health at the district level, the inspection team consists of 3 Additional District Health Officers and 16 supervisors. Secondly, Apart from this the Chief Executive Officer appoints a Flying Squad, which can visit and inspect the work of any department within the district. Thirdly, a flying squad is randomly appointed by the Deputy Director, Akola and visits the district health offices falling in the purview of Akola division of Maharashtra state. Fourthly, the Additional Director of Health Services, Family Welfare Bureau, Pune also visits the health department and inspects the work being undertaken.

The research study is an impact assessment of communication strategies applied through the public health department in the rural (tribal) areas and hence comes under the jurisdiction of the District Health Office, Amravati.

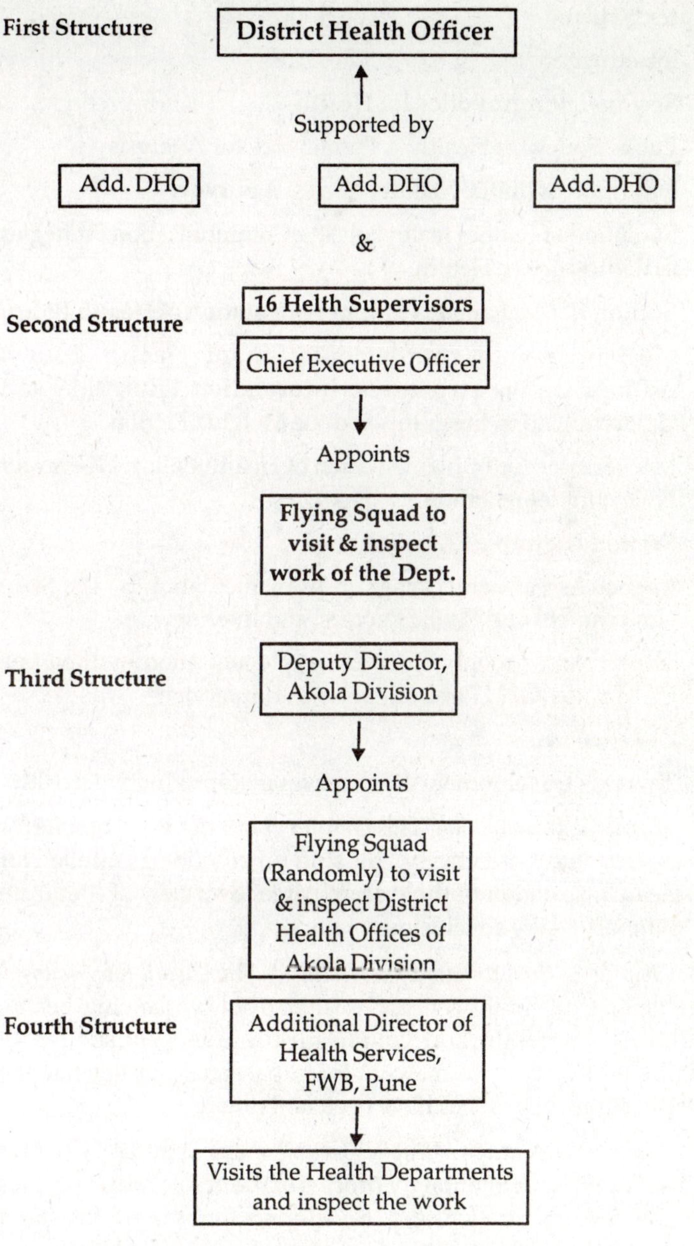
First Structure
District Health Officer
Supported by
Add. DHO
Add. DHO
Add. DHO
&
16 Helth Supervisors
Second Structure
Chief Executive Officer
Appoints
Flying Squad to visit & inspect work of the Dept.
Third Structure
Deputy Director, Akola Division
Appoints
Flying Squad (Randomly) to visit & inspect District Health Offices of Akola Division
Fourth Structure
Additional Director of Health Services, FWB, Pune
Visits the Health Departments and inspect the work

Diagram – 1.1

Chapter Scheme

I. Introduction

Section I: Public Policy for Health

II. Public Policy for Health: A Framework for Analysis

III. Evolution of Public Health Policies: A Survey

IV. Evolution of Public Health Policies: Communication Strategies in Reproductive Health

Section II: Mechanisms for Implementation of Health Policy

V. Mechanisms for Implementation of Health Policy: Administrative structures; Information Education and Communication Programs and the Melghat Region

VI. Mechanisms for Implementation of Health Policy: NGOs and Policy Implementation

Section III: Impact Assessment

VII. Impact Assessment: Program Implementation by the State Government and Public Reports, and Interview

VIII. Impact Assessment: Program Implementation by the State Government and Public Reports, and Interview

Conclusion

IX. Towards Development Alternatives in Reproductive Health

Chapter 1. Introduction. This chapter spells out the rationale for this research study, objectives of the study, methodology applied for the research, selection of the research area, overview of literature and summary of the conclusions of the study.

Chapter 2. Public Policy for Health: A Framework for Analysis. This chapter explains the concepts related to policy, planning, health, Reproductive Health and communication and subsequently provides with a policy framework for impact analysis. Further, the criteria for impact analysis have been laid down.

Chapter 3. Evolution of Public Health Policies: A Survey. Chapter 3 focuses upon the evolutionary process of the public health policies in India, referring to the pre-independence and the post independence efforts consisting of National policies for Health and

Population, planning process in the five year plans, the recommendations of the health committees and commissions and its implementation, the participation of India in international conferences and the policy changes after the participation in International Conference on Population and Development in 1994.

Chapter 4. Evolution of Public Health Policies: Communication Strategies in Reproductive Health. The focus of this chapter is on the policies related to Reproductive Health in general and health education and communication strategies applied in the field of Reproductive Health in particular.

Chapter 5 and 6: Mechanisms for Implementation of Health Policy. The second section focuses on the following: (i) The administrative structures of the Central and Maharashtra State Government for implementation of Public Health programs. (ii) The Public Health schemes implemented by the Maharashtra State Government, with special reference to the Melghat region of Amravati district. (iii) The selected efforts made by various nongovernmental organizations (NGOs) in advocacy at policy and implementation levels.

Chapter 7 and 8: Impact Assessment. This section focuses upon the Melghat Region with the emphasis on the crisis of infant mortality in 1993, which led to a series of studies about the efficacy of various government programs in Public Health Policy and the emergence of new approaches to tackle the situation. Secondly, it covers the impact assessment of the new policies that were implemented after the 1993 crisis.

Chapter 9: Conclusion: Towards Development Alternatives in Reproductive Health. The concluding section presents the findings and the conclusions of the research undertaken.

V. Overview of Literature

Several government documents like policy statements, Five Year Plans, annual reports of the ministries, performance budgets, reports of different committees and commissions have been studied.

Articles from journals, newspapers, books, reviews, working papers, related to Public Health Policy, case studies in Reproductive Health, impact analysis of Public Health Policies from the Reproductive Health angle have been studied. However, from the review of literature, it was revealed, that some remotely similar works have been undertaken, which have been quoted and explained below. The studies were related to effects of failure of communication from the health professionals to the people (as in Gadchiroli study); a policy implication that the Indian government should continue to sponsor family planning messages on radio and television and perhaps even intensify these efforts (as revealed by the National Family Health Survey); requirement of strengthening of IEC component in Maharashtra to reduce the fertility rate (as revealed by the study conducted by Sanjeevani Mulay in Maharashtra); and requirement of database on maternal health status and morbidity, and their correlates; quality of care concerns and women's ability to exercise reproductive choice (as revealed in the study conducted by Shireen Jeejibhoy – Reproductive Health information in India – what are the gaps?); but a study pertaining to impact analysis of communication strategies of Reproductive Health has not been undertaken as yet.

This research study decided to undertake an impact analysis of the communication strategies of Reproductive Health in India, due to the fact that over the past decades there has been a general discrediting of the Indian Family Planning Program. The Reproductive Health approach, however, is not as new as some would claim particularly those who insist that all early Family Planning Programs were totally and blindly demographically driven. Some elements of Reproductive Health were included in earlier formulation of population policies. In fact as early as 1952 the Indian Planning Commission thought Family Planning should be endorsed to improve the health of mothers and children.[4] Apart from this the concept of Health Education was well laid down right from the First Five Year Plan, however the importance of it was gradually realized and accordingly the efforts to emphasize more and more on provision of Information and Education of the people were undertaken.

Due to the changing international trends, it was for the first time that the terminology of Information, Education and Communication (IEC) instead of Health Education was used in the Seventh Five Year Plan[5]. It stated that the progress made so far in the promotion of Health Education is far from satisfactory. Schemes to strengthen health education bureaus, training of medical and paramedical personnel in health education etc., would continue to be implemented with added emphasis. It emphasized upon the efforts for the active use of different types of media to create awareness among the people and motivate them to utilize health services and to adopt healthful practices.

Further, the Ninth Five Year Plan proposed to follow World Bank procedures and assign the work of concurrent evaluation in a few districts on a quarterly basis to specialist communication agencies to assess the impact of IEC in all forms so that the programs could be reoriented on the basis of results of evaluation. Hence it was felt appropriate and necessary to undertake a study, which can reveal the impact occurred due to communication strategies applied in the field of Reproductive Health as a part of implementation of Public Health Policies.

The research study correlates with the following studies identified and theoretical framework from the various books and articles.

1. Bang. R.A. & A.T. Bang[6] explain in a community based study of gynecological problems of rural women in the year 1989 undertaken in Gadchiroli, a remote, backward district in the central part of India determined that the failure of communication was one reason, that the Public Health professionals did not realize the magnitude of gynecological problem that exist. Even though 92% of women had gynecological problems only 7.8% had ever undergone pelvic examination and received any kind of treatment for their reproductive tract infections or any other Reproductive Health problems. This article has helped build the consensus that there is a great requirement to analyze the IEC strategies implemented and measure the impact of it.

2. A study conducted by Robert D Retherford and Vinod Mishra in 1997, reported by National Family Health Survey[7] gave a policy implication that the Indian Government should continue to sponsor family planning messages on radio and television and perhaps even intensify these efforts. This would seem to be a cost-effective approach to reaching the millions of women who are exposed to electronic media and informing

them about the use of contraception and the benefits of small family size. The government should also do what it can to increase general exposure to electronic mass media. The conclusions of this study have encouraged the present research study to go further and analyze the effects of media and messages in the remote tribal parts of the country that lack literacy and lack the reach of electronic media to a large extent.

3. A study conducted by Sanjeevani Mulay[8] shows that despite high contraceptive prevalence in Maharashtra, there is a very moderate decline in birth rate, in the state. Better Reproductive Health facilities leading to reduced foetal losses, lesser childlessness and reduced breast-feeding, can be said to be the main factor contributing in increase in fertility. In such situation, only strengthening of IEC component of the family welfare services can result in decline in fertility in Maharashtra. This has helped research study in building up the case for assessing the impact in tribal areas

4. Shireen Jeejibhoy in a study conducted on – Reproductive Health information in India – what are the gaps?[9] explains that although the NFHS has succeeded in updating and enhancing our data base, it has not been able to address some of the major Reproductive Health issues that lend themselves to being dealt with in large surveys. Among them, maternal health status and morbidity, and their correlates; quality of care concerns and women's ability to exercise reproductive choice are areas where data gaps continue to exist. Women's ability to exercise reproductive choice can only come from the information that she receives and hence it is necessary that first we assess whether the information has reached her and whether there is any impact of the same.

5. Anrudh Jain, in his book, 'Do Population Policies Matter?'[10] looks at policy making as a process, influenced by a number of internal and external factors, guided by the interests of the groups and individuals. It talks of the evolution of policies, involvement of people, influences of internal political systems, international agencies and external financial resources. The author has compared the performance of population policy with the performance of education, health and economic

policies. This comparison explains the effect of factors like political instability or lack of political will on the success or failure of development policy. The book helps in understanding the evolution of public health policies for the research study undertaken and also helps in analyzing the roles of different actors and effects of different strategies applied by the Government of India in the last fifty years.

6. Saroj Pachauri,[11] is one of the paper states that the focus of health programmes should change form a population control approach of reducing numbers to an approach that is gender sensitive and responsive to the Reproductive Health needs of clients. Reproduction Health Programmes should aim to reduce the burden of unplanned and unwanted child bearing and related morbidity and morality. The article reflects that to date, the impact of Family Planning Programmes has been measured mainly in terms of their contribution to increased contraceptive prevalence and decreased fertility. These indicators are inadequate for measuring the impact of Reproductive Health Programmes and hence new indicators from the perspective of the client are urgently needed.

7. K. Srinivasan, in his book Regulating reproduction in India's population – efforts, results and recommendations[12], explains the nature of efforts that have been put into the Indian Family Planning Program, the results achieved at the state and national level and the implications of successful experiences. It reflects upon the concern for regulating reproduction, it however correlates how each of the policy based on this had its concerns in improving maternal health and reduction of maternal mortality and morbidity.

8. Margaret Catley Carlson in her article[13] talks about the lasting impact of International Conference on Population and Development (ICPD), Cairo, in many countries. It explains about the two important messages that were crafted at this conference – the importance of Reproductive Health and a new emphasis on the empowerment of women. While Cairo Conference recognized that contraception and Family Planning are necessary components of any Reproductive Health program, it signaled that the world had to complete the

paradigm shift with respect to the way the contraceptives should be provided: no longer to achieve any targets but to offer a range of good quality service to meet the specific needs of the individual.

9. Subhash Kashyap, in his book National Policy Studies[14] presents factual and objective explanation on the evolution of National Health policy 1983 and reflects upon the conditions and causes of its formulation.

10. R.S. Ganpathy and others in their book Public Policy and Policy Analysis in India,[15] focus on the operational problems of the public programs leading to the increasing realization that our research must encompass the analysis of policy options and assumptions as there is a close link between the public policy process, policy choice and implementation. It explains on the evolution of Public Health Policies in India and implementation processes through practical case studies.

11. Shepard Forman and Romita Ghosh[16], in their book reflect upon the Reproductive Health approach endorsed at the ICPD as the one which has permeated policies and programs to varying degrees in many countries, although the language of Reproductive Health has entered Population and Family Planning discourse, in some countries, the population growth continues to dominate the Population and Family Planning Policy. The developing country case studies presented in the book reveal important advances in policy formulation, financing, and delivery of services in the health and population sectors. However, they underscore that more needs to be accomplished, especially in improving the Reproductive Health care of women, men and adolescents as well as improving access to information and quality health care services.

12. The Government of India document entitled "National Population Policy, 2000"[17] (NPP 2000) affirms the commitment of Government towards voluntary and informed choice and consent and citizens while availing of Reproductive Heath Care Services, and continuation and target free approach in administering Family Planning Services. The NPP 2000 provides a policy framework for advancing goals and

prioritizing strategies during the next decade to meet the Reproductive and Child Health needs of the people of India. The National Population Policy 2000, which has been influenced thoroughly by the ICPD and its Program of Action (POA), has laid down each and every aspect of Reproductive Health. The focus on the tools and strategies to be applied for the implementation of effective programs in Reproductive Health is explicit.

13. The Government of India document, entitled "Manual on Community Needs Assessment Approach on Family Welfare Program"[18], assesses the achievements of the Family Welfare Program on the basis of the targets given from above for individual contraceptives, it further explains that this led to a situation where the achievement of contraceptive targets had become ends in themselves. The top down target approach was started with the supposition that the achievement of contraceptive targets somewhat would definitely lead to a decrease in birth rate and subsequently in decrease in population. However, over the years, it became apparent that there were numerous drawbacks in the top down target approach. Hence with the removal of targets in 1997, the new program of RCH was launched on the basis of drawbacks and problems identified through the CNA approach.

14. The Government of India document entitled "Reproductive and Child Health Program"[19], incorporates the components covered under the Child Survival and Safe Motherhood (CSSM) Program and includes two additional components, on relating to sexually transmitted diseases (STD) and other relating to reproductive tract infections (RTI). The importance of IEC activity cannot be overstated for demystifying the RCH and population issues among public and in advocacy role. Imaginatively produced programs have a very strong persuasive effect. Therefore, the Department of Family Welfare has been implementing a large IEC program under which extensive use is being made of Doordarshan, All India Radio, Directorate of Advertising and Visual Publicity, Directorate of Field publicity, Song and Drama division and Films Division under the Ministry of Information and Broadcasting. In

addition, Mahila Swasthya Sanghs, sensitization of opinion leaders, health awareness units in Nehru Yuvak Kendras are being supported. It is proposed to follow World Bank procedures and assign the work of concurrent evaluation in a few districts every quarter to specialist communication agencies to assess the impact of IEC in all forms so that the programs could be reoriented on the basis of results of evaluation.

15. An eight-country study by USAID[20] reflects upon the intensified worldwide focus on Reproductive Health Policies and Programs after the ICPD held in Cairo. The case studies show that within their unique social, cultural and programmatic contexts, countries like India have made significant progress in placing Reproductive Health on the national health agenda. Policy dialogue has occurred and that considerable progress is achieved in broadening participation in Reproductive Health Policy making.

16. The case study by Dileep Mavlankar, Rani Bang & Abhay Bang[21] reflects upon the work of "SEARCH", a non-governmental organization working in the field of Reproductive Health in the rural India. The approaches, methods, skills and experiences that are important for proper implementation in the field of Reproductive Health have been laid down.

17. Phyllis Tilson Piotrow and others in their book[22] talk about the application of communication study as a powerful force for public education and behaviour change in the last fifty years. With the growth of mass media and the scientific methods to measure its impact, communication now plays a crucial role in social change. It promises to play an even larger role in the future.

18. Phyllis Tilson Piotrow & Jose G. Rimon II in their article[23] reflect upon the learning and knowledge curve shifting from agriculture to public health in the last quarter of the century, the increasing prominence of the issues such as Population and Family Planning, Primary Health Care, Maternal and Child Health, and other diseases, has focused attention on the role of communication in Public Health Programs. The article talks

about the Indian case study of a strategic campaign centered around the slogan "Come let's talk" in Uttar Pradesh, the largest state of India. Formative communication strategy research identified the lack of open discussion about Family Planning and other modern methods as a key inhibitor amongst all intended audiences.

Proceeding from the Constitution, we have had several Five-Year plan documents each of which contains tour d'horizon of social and economic policies that are proposed for pursuit in the relevant plan period. Given their basically documentational character, the plans have provided steady grist to many academic mills in India. A whole body of policy analysis in the country is addressed to policy continuities, contradictions, slippages and graduation in the language of the plans and to issues relating to promises vis a vis performance[24].

VI. A Summary of Conclusions

The conclusions of this study are in two parts. One relates to the findings based on the study of Melghat region and the other to general observations that follow from the case study.

The findings of the Survey of Melghat Region are as Follows:

- Causes of infant mortality deaths – generally illness and weakness are the responses, however, no specific cause is known.
- Reproductive Health problems – mostly white discharge, abdominal pain and Sexually Transmitted Diseases, lack of nutrition also leading to natural abortions amongst these women is a common factor.
- In case of Reproductive Health problems women generally approach the ANM or Dai.
- People talked about various sources of communication and are getting information about Reproductive Health through radio, street plays, posters etc, but have also quoted the language problem, that is the language of communication is Marathi, whereas the spoken language of Korkus is Hindi and Korku.

- Women have demanded that the communicators should talk to the men in their households regarding their Reproductive Health problems.
- Out of the 87 beneficiaries receiving benefits – most of them have received partly money and partly medicines in Matrutva Anudan Yojana and are aware of the nutritional requirements of a pregnant woman.
- Despite this, most of the women have felt satisfied about the benefits from the schemes.

The contents of the policies have been studied and it is found that the policies are ambitious, comprehensive and serve as models. In this study the researcher has made the following observations with regards to the implementation of Public Health Policies in the field of Reproductive Health:

- Target oriented programs have less focus on voluntarism
- Family Planning is the key aspect of all the policies with a strong bias towards sterilization, despite the cafeteria approach.
- Lack of involvement of any other ministry apart from the Health Ministry.
- Program is formulated and funded by the Central Government, but implementation relies heavily on health facility run by the State Government.
- Theoretically, states are encouraged to modify the program according to their needs; however, in reality it does not happen.
- The top down command approach of the program undermines the ownership of the program by local authorities.
- Exaggeration of performance by the program officials.
- Lack of emphasis on male participation and male responsibility.
- Lack of understanding about the socioeconomic problems faced by the health workers.
- Camp approach – lacking in counseling or information about other options.

Similarly, the researcher has made the following observations with regards to the application of communication strategies and education programs in the field of Reproductive Health:

- Dramatic increase in expansion of physical infrastructure but not in training or educational material.
- People's education is the weakest link in the impact of the program.
- Limited reach of mass media, radio has the broadest reach, next limited reach television or movies, low literacy rate-even more limited reach of print media.
- People responsible for public education are not professionally trained.
- No proper audio-visual equipments at the PHC
- Absence of education material in PHC other than regular posters.
- Public education efforts not providing for adequate information, for example the government sponsored media campaign for the birth control pill said "See a Doctor" giving the message that the pill is unsafe.
- Low funds for advertising and social marketing.
- Education material culturally inappropriate and lacking in audience orientation.

Experts presenting evidence in many countries, suggest that mass media are not only legitimizing and stimulating discussion but also are triggering behaviour change. Impressive results have been reported from campaigns using radios. A considerable number of survey respondents said information from the mass media motivated their clinic visits.

In the Field of Public Health Substantial Evidence Shows that:

1. People want to know more about their health;
2. People want to talk more about health to friends and family members, hear about it through mass media and discuss it with competent health care providers;

3. People are willing to change their health behaviour; and
4. Public Health communication programs are helping people make these changes.

A thorough evaluation of the impact of communication strategies includes an analysis of its indirect as well as direct effects on health behaviour. Because it is generally observed that:

- At all levels people lack information.
- Even if they have information they have no knowledge about how to use it.
- Even if they apply this information with understanding, they do not know of its advantages, disadvantages and complications.
- And even if they know of complications, how to tackle these complications is the last thing that they know of.

REFERENCES

1. Details Taken from the *1991 Census, Amravati District, Maharashtra, 1991.*
2. Information Procured from *DHO office, Amravati District, Maharashtra, 2003.*
3. Lok Arogya Margdarshan Pratishthan, Melghat Mitra, and Peoples Rural Education Movement (PREM) are Some *NGOs Working in the Melghat Region.*
4. Anrudh Jain, *Do Population Policies Matter?-Fertility and Politics in Egypt, India, Kenya and Mexico.* (New York, Population Council, 1998) p. 12.
5. Government of India, Seventh Five Year Plan, (New Delhi, Planning Commission 1985).
6. Bang. R.A., A.T. Bang, et al. High Prevalence of Gynecological Diseases in Rural Indian Women. *Lancet* 1(8629): 85-88, 1989.
7. Robert D Retherford and Vinod Mishra, 'Media Exposure Increases Contraceptive Use', *National Family Health Survey,* (Bulletin No. 7, 1997).
8. Sanjeevani Mulay, 'Demographic Transition in Maharashtra, 1980-1993', *Economic and Political Weekly,* 34(42 & 43) 3063-3074. 1999.
9. Shireen Jeejibhoy, 'Reproductive Health Information in India – What are the Gaps?', *Economic and Political Weekly,* 34(42&43) 3075-3080, 1999.
10. Anrudh Jain, n. 4.
11. Saroj Pachauri, *Definng a Reproductive Health Package for India: A Proposed Framework, South and East Asia*– Regional Working Papers, (New Delhi. The Population Council, 1995).

12. K. Srinivasan, *Regulating Reproduction in India's Population – Efforts, Results and Recommendations*. (New Delhi. Sage Publications, 1995.)

13. Margaret Catley Carlson. *From Cairo to Kayoro – Bringing Reproductive Health to a Village in Ghana*, (New York. The Population Council, 1999).

14. Subhash Kashyap, *National Policy Studies*, (The Lok Sabha Secretariat, New Delhi, India, Tata McGraw-Hill Publishing Company Limited, 1990).

15. R.S. Ganpathy, S.R. Ganesh, Rushikesh Maru, Samuel Paul, Ram Mohan Rao, *Public Policy and Policy Analysis in India*, (New Delhi, Sage Publications, 1985.)

16. Shepard Forman and Romita Ghosh, *Promoting Reproductive Health-Investing in Health for Development*, (London. Lynne Rienner Publishers, 2000).

17. Government of India, *National Population Policy 2000*, (New Delhi, Department of Family Welfare, Government of India, 2000).

18. Government of India, *Manual on Community Needs Assessment Approach in Family Welfare Program*, (New Delhi, Ministry of Health and Family Welfare, Government of India, 1998).

19. Government of India, *Reproductive and Child Health Program*, (New Delhi, Ministry of Health and Family Welfare, Government of India, 1997).

20. Karen Hardee, Kokila Agarwal, Nancy Luke, Ellen Wilson, Margaret Pendzich, Marguerite Farrell, Harry Cross, *Post Cairo Reproductive Health Policies and Programs – A Comparative Study of Eight Countries*, (Washington DC, USAID, 1998).

21. Dileep Mavlankar, Rani Bang, Abhay Bang, *Quality Reproductive Health Services in Rural India*, (India. International Council on Management of Population Programs, 1998).

22. Phyllis Tilson Piotrow, D. Lawrence Kincaid, Jose G. Rimon II, & Ward Rinehart, *Health Communication – Lessons from Family Planning and Reproductive Health* (Johns Hopkins School of Public Health, Praeger Publishers, 1997).

23. Phyllis Tilson Piotrow & Jose G. Rimon II, 'Asia's Population and Family Planning Programs: Leaders in Strategic Communication', *Asia-Pacific Population Journal*, Vol. 14, No. 4 1999, p. 73-90.

24. R.S. Ganpathy et al. n. 15. p. 257.

2

Public Policy for Health

A Theoretical Framework

Introduction

The present chapter looks at the concepts related to policy: viz. planning, formulation, implementation, impact and analysis. Concepts related to health: viz. reproductive health, information education and communication are explained and a policy framework for impact analysis is presented. Further, the criteria for impact analysis have been laid down.

I. Concepts of Policy-Planning, Formulation, Implementation and Analysis

Definition of Policy

Policy is often treated as embracing a set sequence of decisions used by some to distinguish decisions about a particular governmental action, goals or preferences. Public policy may be expressed in a variety of forms, including laws, local ordinances, court decisions, executive order, decisions of administrators, or even unwritten understanding of what is to be done. "Policy " without the modifier "public" is sometimes regarded as synonymous with governmental decision.

Public Policy

Public policy as a separate discipline originated in the West. Donoughue and Klitgaard review experiences in the UK, the USA and the other developing countries.[1] It could be said that public policies are those policies, which are public in nature. They are formulated and implemented by the authority in a political system, which aim at the fulfillment of certain specific goals for the betterment of society.

Policy Planning and Formulation

Planning is essentially an attempt at working out a rational solution of problems, an attempt to co-ordinate means and ends; it is thus different from the traditional hit-and-miss methods by which 'reforms' and 'reconstruction' are often undertaken. It follows that a considerable part of the planning authority's task is to assess the significance of some of these indeterminate or partially known factors at work in the life of the community and to recommend policies on the best judgment available. This is particularly so in India today. The function of the Central Government is to evolve a national plan, to work out a coordinated policy for implementation of the same, to watch and assess the progress of major development schemes in the different parts of the country, and to constantly initiate and promote action in furtherance of the objectives and targets defined[2].

Public policy making is a complex process, which has a number of governmental agencies and actors and non-governmental agencies and actors playing an important role. Any policy is formulated to attain some goals and objectives. The outputs of a policy making process are the results which come through in the form of one policy or the other. Efforts to increase level of literacy, health for all, better roads, effective delivery system etc are the outputs of some of the policies. The outcome of these outputs in the form of policies is the impact of the policies.

In India, the Parliament is the supreme policy making body. The policies enacted and implemented need to be in conformity with the Constitutional provisions. In case it is not so, the policy may be declared as void. The Judiciary is empowered to strike down a subordinate or administrative legislation in case it is ultra vires of the Constitution, it violates the Constitution, and it runs counter to the enabling Act's provisions. The Judiciary also controls the activities of the Legislature and Executive through its power of Judicial Review. Through this the courts have the powers to declare acts of legislative and executive branches as unconstitutional. It is based on the assumption that the Constitution is the supreme law and any action or act, which is contrary to the constitution, is void.

Policy Implementation

Unless and until the policies formulated are executed in fair, impartial, and effective way howsoever good the policy intents may be, the expected results can never be attained. The Legislature and Judiciary have an important role to play in implementation of the policies. Implementation as a process is translated into working through institutions and agencies, which are assigned the said task of execution of a specific policy. Besides planning, the hierarchical levels and elements of control are essential ingredients of the work mechanism of implementation. Implementation proceeds through several stages, commencing with policy outputs or decisions of the implementing agencies, which included the translation of statutory objectives into a substantive regulations and standards operating procedures.

Agencies of Implementation

Most of the activity surrounding policy implementation takes place within the administrative or bureaucratic agencies. The implementation of policies is largely done by the bureaucrats as they have control over the resources and legal powers of the government. They are passed on directives to implement the policies by the three organs of the government, that is, Executive, Legislature and Judiciary. It is also commonly felt that the political executive who are the elected representatives of the people in democracies perform the major task of implementing the policies.

Policy implementation is the major job obligation of the permanent executive. Of course the political executive also has it in its task performance zone. Certain non- governmental agencies like citizens, interest groups, voluntary organizations etc. also have a role to play in policy implementation.

Policy Process and Policy Impact

Once the policy is formulated, with the contribution of both governmental and non- governmental agencies, it is put to execution.

At the stage of policy implementation also, various channels and agencies are involved in its work for achieving the stated objectives of the policy. The outputs of the policy bring to light certain outcomes, which in other words could be said as the impact of the policy.

Policy impact is of crucial importance in the overall policymaking process. The impact of the policy whether direct or indirect, immediate or futuristic, symbolic or tangible is ascertained and measured through the process of policy evaluation. Policy evaluation as a process is as old as policy making itself. It is a means of getting the policy makers the relevant information and knowledge regarding a policy problem, about the relative purposefulness and effectiveness of past and prevailing strategies for addressing, reducing or eliminating the problem, and regarding the observed effectiveness of specific policies.

Policies are goal oriented and aim at the betterment of the society. Policy evaluation plays its role not only after the formulation and implementation of the policy but its starts right from the identification of various issues for making policies and putting these on policy agenda after viewing the various alternatives from different angles and thus selecting the ones best required in accordance with the need of time and society.

Policy Analysis

Policy analysis is a comparatively recent phenomenon in public systems. Its origin was in the United States in the sixties, and in India it is began to come into vogue in eighties. The growth of policy analysis has been characterized by the application of prevalent methodologies in social science enquiry and research. This parallels the growth of methodology in natural sciences over the last three hundred years. This has been a positivist tradition that has made enormous efforts to attain the status of the natural sciences for social science through rigorous, precise and analytic methodologies. The domination of the empirical method in social science and its application in policy analysis clearly reflects these efforts[3].

Policy analysis refers to an explicit, focused, systematic analysis of the outputs of governments and their effects on society. "process studies of congressional committees, public opinion, party competition, and so forth, are not considered policy analysis unless the linkage to political outputs is made explicit[4].

Policy analysis has become a professionalized technical activity. The main task facing the policy analyst is of developing an indigenous craft of public policy analysis, which is at once useful in solving practical problems and sensitive to social structural issues. Of-course no policy analysis research can be rendered useful unless policy makers recognize analysis as an important aid to decision making. A climate of mutual trust and understanding between policy makers and policy analysts can be forged through integrated programs involving research, training and consultation[5].

There is a common, often unstated, assumption that policy analysis improves policymaking. In recent years this has been challenged in a radical way. The connections between theory and practice, knowledge and action are very tenuous and in the field of policy making they are even more so. There is considerable evidence that policy analysis is a fairly minor determinant of policy making. Other more important determinants are (a) the context (b) the leadership (c) politics of bureaucracy, interest groups, and legislatures and (d) public images the media generates about the policy issues. The conventional diffusion model of policy research implies that the research gets translated into practice (instrumental use of knowledge). This diffusion model typically focuses on a single, rational decision maker and represents by and large the middle class interests in preserving status quo social order and in making incremental changes. Work in different t contexts indicates that this model is not realistic. In the words of Paul Feyerabend, "there are no data or facts independent of prior theory that organizes them[6]". This poses very clearly what one would describe as the theory-facts dilemma, that is to say, choice among competing theories need to be based on empirical dta. However, such data itself is dependent on a prior theoretical framework. The political use of policy research for postponing decisions and to justify decisions already made, are very well known. Again the question of interests looms large in the utilization of policy analysis.[7]

Policy analysis in India, while relatively uncommon in the form it is known in the United States, has been undertaken in a variety of ways. Our constitution and legislation make policy pronouncements and our Five Year Plans involve a good deal of analysis about resource allocation and investment decisions. Several committees and government statements in the form of white papers, resolutions, etc., include a good deal of analysis of different policies. Most of the programs that have been started are based on some kind of policy analysis. The methods that are used are of various kinds: economic modeling, optimization studies, social cost-benefit analysis, micro economic analysis, survey research and input – output models. As one can see readily, there is a domination of economics in such policy analyses, and the economists largely dominate the Planning Commission and the Ministry of Finance in this area[8].

Updating of Policy

Each and every policy that is formulated and implemented is updated/modified from time to time as per the requirements of changing scenarios.

II. Concepts of Health, Reproductive Health and Communication

Health

The concise Oxford Dictionary defines health as the state of soundness of body or mind. Health according to the World Health Organization (WHO) is a state complete physical, mental, and social well being and not merely the absence of disease or deformity[9].

Public Health

Health, however always remained an area to be looked after and taken care of by family guidance, personal care, individual choice, and socio religious norms. In fact only recently the evolution of the concept of public health has encouraged the state and the society to regulate individual private behavior related to ones health for the good of the whole. It is only in this century the public efforts have been organized to meet their own needs to protect the individual's health. Today the Public Health Programs include the national and international programs to address the health and demographic concerns, to promote safe motherhood, to increase child survival, to cure tuberculosis, to stop the spread of HIV/ AIDS and other sexually transmitted diseases.[10]

In more concrete terms public health can be defined as "the planning, carrying out and evaluation of health measures and system services that both maintain and improve the health of a population group and prevent and control disease within that population group"

A further enlargement of the concept of health has been postulated as community health. Community health, whether applied to individual or community, is applied to achieve such a well being that one may function at the optimum level not as an individual but also as a useful member of the social groups and the community.

Reproductive Health

Considering the efforts being made in the field of Public Health, human reproduction has always been an important issue to be looked at from the point of individual's choice and socio religious norms. In the past few years it has emerged as one of the most sensitive and challenging areas of Public Health. The seventies and eighties saw a shift towards the qualitative aspects of growth, including investments in education, health care, clean water, and sanitation. As a result of this development at international level, the UN sponsored international conferences of the nineties reflected and reinforced the evolution of this development thinking. These included: the well being of children – 1990; a Clean Healthy and Sustainable Environment –1992; Universality of Human Rights – 1993; Reproductive Health and Population – 1994; Social Development 1995; Women's Rights – 1995; Safe and Productive habitats – 1996; and Food Security – 1996; formulating a platform for sustainable development for the century to come.[11]

The United Nation's 1994 International Conference on Population and Development (ICPD) held in Cairo, Egypt was a landmark in the field of population and development. The rejection of the concept of family control and recognition that smaller families and slower population growth can be achieved through free choice and by ensuring the conditions that encourage such choice was undertaken. The Reproductive Health approach embodied in the ICPD Program of Action (POA) emphasized and stressed the importance of advancing gender equality, equity, the empowerment of women and the women's ability to control their own fertility.

ICPD defines Reproductive Health as "a state of complete physical, mental and social well being and not merely the absence of disease or infirmity, in all matters relating to the reproductive system and its functions and processes. Reproductive Health therefore implies that people have the capability to reproduce and the freedom to decide if, when and how often to do so. Implicit in this last condition are the rights of men and women to be informed and to have access to safe, effective, affordable and acceptable methods of family planning of their choice, as well as other methods of their choice for regulation of fertility which are not against the law, and the right of access to appropriate health care services that will enable women to go safely through pregnancy and childbirth and provide couples with the best chance of having a healthy infant". In line with the above definition of reproductive health, reproductive health care is defined as the constellation of methods, techniques, and services, which contribute to Reproductive Health and well being through preventing and solving Reproductive Health problems. It also includes sexual health, the purpose of which is the enhancement of life and personal relations, and not merely counseling and care related to reproduction and sexually transmitted diseases. (ICPD – 94) [12]

The definition of Reproductive Health as spelt out by ICPD promotes women's involvement in the planning, management, implementation and evaluation of Reproductive Health programs and emphasizes the role of men as active partners in the family planning and family life. It recommends that primary healthcare systems in all countries should provide a range of Reproductive Health information and services including but not limited to family planning. Consequently, communication is critical for ensuring women's empowerment in the field of Reproductive Health through their participation.

Communication

The spread and practice of all the concerned programs in the field of public health have been making efforts to change the individual and social behavior. Communication has been the most crucial aspect in bringing about the social change.

Communication has been defined as all those planned or unplanned processes through which one person influences the behaviour of other persons. From this standpoint, communication is the science of interaction between individuals, which has behavioural consequences[13]. The Concise Oxford Dictionary defines communication as the science and the practice of transmitting information. Communication, as a discipline developed from Sociology, Social Psychology and Political Science. Initially it was applied only in the schools of Journalism and Speech. Today it is being applied and has advanced as an important field in public health. Every national and international health program consists of communication components with a staff and a budget for the same. Communication thus aims to play a major role and influence the decision making at all levels, be it personal, family, community, mass media or at the national policy making level. Communication results in the spread of knowledge, values, social norms, disadvantages and advantages of certain practices.

The power of communication today stems from two recent developments, the rapid growth of communication media and the notable increase in our understanding of the communication process. With regards to reproductive health, communication is the key process underlying changes in the knowledge of the means of contraception, in attitudes toward fertility control, use of contraceptives, and in the openness of local cultures to new ideas and aspirations and new health behaviour[14].

Messages related to Reproductive Health of women in general and Family Planning in particular represent a major shift in individual and social behaviour. Communication has been crucial to this shift. Listening to the discussions of formerly taboo topics, such as some aspects of reproductive health, in community meetings, and on television and radio can encourage them to open up and talk with friends and family members.

III. A Framework for Policy Analysis

The basic idea of the research is to look at the different Public Health Policies enacted by the Government of India since its independence so as to understand the significant steps and measures taken by the government in achieving quality Reproductive Health for the women of the country and undertaking impact analysis of communication strategies used for implementing these policies effectively.

For undertaking the research study, the understanding of theoretical and conceptual aspects of policy planning, formulation, implementation, analysis and impact is critical. Further, from the perspective of health dimensions it is required to understand the conceptual background of General Health, Public Health and Reproductive Health. The need for understanding the concept of communication and its growing and changing trends leading to the holistic concept of Information, Education and Communication (IEC) is also a critical part of the study.

Hence, firstly, the research study looks at the planning, formulation, implementation and carries out an impact assessment of various Public Health Programs and Schemes in India. The planning process since the time of independence and its continuation in each and every Five Year Plan, the formulation processes and stages of the National Health Policy and the National Population Policy with the involvement of different committees and commissions are studied in order to gather the focus laid on the aspects of Reproductive Health in each of this attempt. Further the contents of the various programs based on the abovementioned policies and the initial National Family Planning Program is also studied in order to analyze the importance paid to the aspects of Reproductive Health. Various internal as well as external factors influencing the nature of the health policies, programs and policy implementation are also analyzed.

Secondly, the research study focuses on the changed and broader concept of Reproductive Health from what it was earlier referred to as Maternal Health. It goes by the present day concept of Reproductive Health which is holistic in nature and consists of several aspects of the complete span of reproductive age, be it details related to reproductive cycle, age at marriage, results of early child bearing, unwanted pregnancies, unsafe abortions, importance of institutional deliveries, reproductive tract infections, sexually transmitted diseases, or even the family planning methods.

Thirdly, the research study looks at the importance of Health Education in the field of Reproductive Health with the newly developed concept of Information, Education and Communication (IEC). It tries to study the communication strategies applied by the government as a part of the implementation of policies in order to spread more knowledge and information regarding Reproductive Health. The details on communication strategies being looked at for impact analysis are regarding the method of communication, the sources of communication, the language used, the place where the information is provided etc. which reveal the efforts undertaken by the government (in effective implementation of its policies) to provide the client with required information.

The government policies formulate a number of need based schemes to be extended to the clients for attainment of better health. The research study also focuses on these area specific schemes extended to the couples in reproductive age so as to provide them with better and quality health. Here the impact analysis tries to assess the knowledge and information level of the communicator (both the policy maker, the implementer and the actual communicator that is the grass root level staff) as well as that of the client to whom this information or scheme is extended.

The data is collected from the tribal and remote parts of Amravati district of Maharashtra. It is important to notice why this particular area is selected to assess the impact of communication strategies in Reproductive Health. This is so because the area is known for its extensive health inputs and measures undertaken by the Government of Maharashtra, especially since the year 1993, when the area was struck with the problem of Protein Energy Malnutrition and caused a number of infantile deaths. The measures undertaken included a number of schemes and programs to reduce malnutrition and infant as well as maternal mortality. The people from the area are illiterate, extremely poor, unable to afford any external luxuries, with a primitive culture and cut away from the mainstream. The success of any policy is determined by its reach. This being a tribal area, the relevance and impact of the Reproductive Health policy should be assessed in terms of whether it has reached the remotest regions and the marginalized sections of the society that is the tribal people. It was felt more so necessary to study the effects and analyze the impact of any programs or policies implemented in this area, which has not been touched upon by an earlier research study.

Thus the research study tries to utilize the base of conceptual framework of policy analysis in assessing impact of the communication strategies in reproductive health.

IV. Criteria for Impact Analysis

The criteria set for analyzing the impact of various factors being looked at in the research study is as follows:

Criteria for Health in General and Reproductive Health in Particular

- Whether there is provision of essential services for pregnant women?
- Whether there are facilities for prevention, diagnosis and treatment of STDs and RTIs?
- Whether there is an access to contraceptive services and information?
- Whether the facilities for Family Planning are available?
- Whether there exists an emphasis on healthy sexuality – implying control over one's body?
- Whether sexuality education and public awareness on sexual health problems is provided?
- Whether the knowledge of infection free sex and reproduction is extended?
- Whether there exist measures to reduce unintended pregnancies?
- Whether there is access to safe abortion and post abortion care?
- Whether there exists access to care in obstetric emergencies?
- Whether the measures to improve the quality of maternity care have been undertaken?

Criteria for Program and Policy Success

- Whether the implementers are well qualified for their jobs?
- Whether the personnel implementing the programs/policies have received relevant and adequate training?

- Whether the work profile of the personnel is clear and adequate?
- Whether the personnel are aware of the existing government schemes?
- Whether they have a clear role in implementation of government schemes?
- Whether there exists adequate infrastructural facility in the village?
- Whether the personnel have any suggestion regarding improvement of these facilities?
- Whether adequate attention is being given to the health factor?
- Whether the government policies regarding health relevant and adequate?
- Whether the government schemes related to health relevant and adequate?
- Whether there exist any specific schemes related to reproductive health of women?
- Whether the personnel face any problem in disseminating information about these schemes?
- Whether the problems faced by people related to these government schemes are critical?
- Whether the problems faced by personnel in disseminating information about these schemes are considered?
- Whether the social problems faced by the personnel while doing work related to schemes is considered?
- Whether the reasons for low awareness of people regarding the government facilities and schemes are known by the personnel?
- Whether government measures have been taken to improve these facilities and quality of services?

Criteria for Communication Strategies (IEC)

- Whether there exist strategies for communication?
- What are these strategies?

- Who are the personnel involved in implementation of these strategies?
- Whether all the communication and schemes extended to the people are within their reach?
- Whether these strategies and schemes are adequate?
- Are these strategies and schemes relevant?
- Do these strategies and schemes possess clarity?
- Are these strategies and schemes precise?
- Whether there exist adequate structures to implement these strategies and schemes?
- Whether adequate budget is available for its implementation? And
- Whether these strategies have resulted in any behavioural or attitudinal change?

REFERENCES

1. R.S. Ganpathy, S.R. Ganesh, Rushikesh Maru, Samuel Paul, Ram Mohan Rao, Public Policy and Policy Analysis in India, New Delhi, India, Sage Publications, 1985. p. 9.

2. Government of India, Chapter 1 – Planning – First Five Year Plan, New Delhi, Planning Commission 1951.

3. R.S. Ganpathy, S.R. Ganesh, Rushikesh Maru, Samuel Paul, Ram Mohan Rao, Public Policy and Policy Analysis in India, New Delhi, India, Sage Publications, 1985. p. 30.

4. Susan B. Hansen, Public Policy Analysis Some Recent Development and Current Problems, Chapter No 08.

5. R.S. Ganpathy, S.R. Ganesh, Rushikesh Maru, Samuel Paul, Ram Mohan Rao, Public Policy and Policy Analysis in India, New Delhi, India, Sage Publications, 1985. Pg. No. 9.

7. R.S. Ganapthy, On Methodologies for Policy Analysis, Indian Institute Of Management, Ahmedabad, W.P. No:- 481, October:- 1983 Page No:- 24, 25, 26 & 27.

8. R.S. Ganapthy, On Methodologies for Policy Analysis, Indian Institute Of Management, Ahmedabad, W.P. No:- 481, October:- 1983 Page No:-24, 25, 26 & 27.

9. Quoted in Subhash Kashyap, National Policy Studies, (The Lok Sabha Secretariat, New Delhi, India, Tata McGraw-Hill Publishing Company Limited, 1990.) p. 377.

10. Phyllis Tilson Piotrow, D. Lawrence Kincaid, Jose G. Rimon II, & Ward Rinehart, Health Communication – Lessons from Family Planning and Reproductive Health, Johns Hopkins School of Public Health, USA, Praeger Publishers, 1997. Pg. No. 9.

11. Shepard Forman and Romita Ghosh, Promoting Reproductive Health-Investing in Health for Development, London, UK, Lynne Rienner Publishers, 2000. Pg. No. 8.

12. Karen Hardee, Kokila Agarwal, Nancy Luke, Ellen Wilson, Margaret Pendzich, Marguerite Farrell, Harry Cross, Post Cairo Reproductive Health Policies and Programs a Comparative Study of Eight Countries, Washington DC, USA. USAID, 1998 Pg. No. 10.

13. Quoted in Phyllis Tilson Piotrow et. al., n. 11.

14. Phyllis Tilson Piotrow, D. Lawrence Kincaid, Jose G. Rimon II, & Ward Rinehart, Health Communication – Lessons from Family Planning and Reproductive Health, Johns Hopkins School of Public Health, USA, Praeger Publishers, 1997. Pg. No. 12.

3

History and Evolution of Health Policies

Background

Introduction

This chapter focuses upon the evolutionary process of the Public Health policies in India, referring to the:

1. Pre-independence and the post independence efforts consisting of National Policies for Health and Population
2. Planning process in the Five Year plans, the recommendations of the Health Committees and Commissions and its implementation
3. The participation of India in international conferences and the policy changes after the participation in International Conference on Population and Development in 1994.

Public Health Policies of India

This study focuses on an impact analysis of the implementation of schemes and programs in the field of Reproductive Health. Family Planning or Population Control historically has been a controversial area for government interventions; hence the policies in the area of Reproductive Health have been couched in acceptable terminology.

Under the Indian Constitution, Health is State subject. The policies are made by the Center and the implementation of the same is the responsibility of the States. Accordingly, the thesis focuses upon the Public Health policies of India and of Maharashtra as the implementation is undertaken by the State Governments.

The initiatives of planning and formulating Public Health policies in India came as a legacy of the British rule, along with the efforts of intelligentsia and the political leaders of the freedom movement. Public Health, though during this period had a lot many issues to study, the concentration was on the increasing population and the causes of infant and maternal mortality and morbidity. Since the independence, the Government of India undertook several attempts and initiatives to launch policies and programs starting from the issues related to population control and family planning. Maternal and Child Health, in this context always remained the priority area. As India went on moving with the agendas and opportunities of the various international conferences held in consecutive decades from that of seventies, the paradigm shift occurred in the year 1994, when India became a signatory to the International Conference on Population and Development (ICPD) held at Cairo, Egypt.

India had traditionally focused on the issues regarding the provision of services and quality care to the men and women of reproductive age-group; implementation of Program of Action (POA) of the ICPD 1994 gave a great boost to the Reproductive Health programs, with principle focus on Health Education through the Information, Education and Communication (IEC) approach.[1] It is in the light of this approach that the present study tries to look at the impact of communication strategies in the field of Reproductive Health. One needs to accept the fact that programs and policies focusing on the Reproductive Health of women have been the most crucial aspects of our Public Health Policy.

I. Pre Independence Period

It was in the nineteen twenties that Prof. R.D. Karve, a lecturer in Mathematics in a Bombay college undertook a life long mission to improve the status of women and advocated widow remarriage and the practice of artificial methods of Family Planning. Being totally devoted to his cause, in 1921 he published a book written in English on birth control and venereal diseases, and in 1927 started a magazine *Samaj Swasthya* (Social Hygiene) in the Marathi language, also started a contraceptive centre in 1921 in Girgaum in the heart of Bombay. Improvement in the status of women in Maharashtra state is largely attributed to the pioneering efforts of Prof. Karve[2].

Unfortunately the birth control program initiated in Bombay and Madras State did not spread very rapidly because of Mahatma Gandhi's strong moral opposition to the use of artificial methods of birth control. He argued that sexual abstinence was the only ethical means of birth control. In spite of the opposition put forward by Gandhi for the use of birth control methods, the women's movement in India through the various voluntary organizations continued to propagandize and support the use of artificial methods of Family Planning.

The British rulers for a long time remained indifferent to Indian problems for two possible reasons, firstly, the British rulers had adopted the policy of non-interference in Indian social matters and as far as possible did not take any measure which could be considered as an intrusion in Indian traditions, customs values and beliefs and secondly, the issue of birth control was controversial in the British home land.

The intellectual foundations laid by Neo Malthusian leagues in various parts of the country and Karve's convincing argument for birth control-mainly that of protecting the health and lives of women led the government of the princely state of Mysore under the enlightened leadership of Maharaja to officially sanction the opening of four Family Planning clinics in 1930[3].

The National Planning Committee (NPC) of the Indian National Congress was set up in 1938. This Committee set up a Sub-Committee on National Health, which made a penetrating assessment of the then existing health situation and health services in the country and recommended measures for their improvement. The Sub-committee submitted an Interim Report in 1940. The remarkable foresight of the Sub-Committee is reflected in the very contemporary tenor of the resolution adopted by the NPC on August 31, 1940 on the basis of this Report. The integration of curative and preventive functions in a single state agency was urged and it was stressed that the maintenance of the health of the people was the responsibility of the State. Significantly, the Final Report of the NPC categorically stated that the cornerstone of the scheme recommended was a '(Community) Health Worker'[4].

The Famine Enquiry Commission appointed by the British Government after the Bengal Famine in its report subtitled to the Central Government contained a section on potential dangers to the economy arising out of rapid population growth especially in a population living in abject poverty and deprived of the bare necessities of life. The commission recommended very strongly that a population control program should become an integral part of any governmental development policy, it also emphasized the need to collect, compile and analyze population related data necessary for developmental assistance to different areas especially compulsory registration of births and deaths. The 1945 recommendations paved the way for the government of India to launch the official program of Family Planning as a part of its developmental strategy immediately after the attainment of independence in 1947.

The second major study that helped to encourage a population policy was the report of the Health Survey and Development Committee also called the Bhore Committee was constituted by the GOI in 1943 under the chairmanship of Sir Joseph Bhore to make a survey of the existing position in regard to health conditions and health organization and to make recommendations for the future developments. The Committee found that they had to confine themselves mainly to statistics of ill-health and death, in the absence of data on positive health[5]. The Committee's 1946 report identified India's major health problems and recommended various measures to improve public health, environmental sanitation, nutrition, and prevention of communicable diseases. It also suggested the organizational structure, most appropriate for implementing these programs. This report devoted an entire chapter to population, strongly recommending the adoption of a National Family Planning Program as an essential Public Health program[6]. The committee considered the deliberate limitation of family size to be "advisable" and noted that it could not be achieved through self-control "to any material extent". The Committee found that nearly half the total numbers of deaths were among children under 10 years of age and in this age group one-half of the mortality took place within the first year of life. The committee found that the low state of public health, as reflected in the high mortality and morbidity (particularly among mothers and children) was preventable and was mainly due to the absence of environmental hygiene, adequate nutrition, adequate preventive and curative health services and intelligent cooperation from the people themselves. To these causes may be added illiteracy, unemployment, poverty, purdah system and early marriages. There was a wide prevalence of in-sanitary conditions in urban and rural areas. The provision for protected water supply and drainage was totally inadequate. Hospitals and dispensaries for providing medical relief to the people, particularly in the rural, areas, were grossly insufficient and the quality of such services was very poor. There were only 0.24 beds per 1,000 population[7].

Some of the important recommendations made by the Committee in their report were: Health services should be placed as close as possible to the people in order to ensure the maximum benefit to the communities to be served. "Health consciousness should be stimulated by providing Health Education on a wide basis as well as by providing opportunities for the individual's participation in local health programs.[8]".

II. Post Independence Period

The efforts in implementing programs and policies related to Reproductive Health began as early as 1952 with the launching of the National Family Planning Program. However in each decade new programs were introduced with a changed focus depending on the influences political or social, within the country or the changes in international scenario. Decade wise changes and evolution of Public Health policies and programs with specific emphasis on Reproductive Health have been accordingly recorded in this chapter.

1950-60

The decade of fifties witnessed the initial vigour in launching of new policies and programs. The very first step was the appointment of Population Policy Committee under Minister of Planning and creation of Family Planning Cell in the office of the Director General of Health Services in April 1950.

Further, in 1952 the program for family limitation and control was launched with the special focus on the health of the mothers and children. The policy document stated the strategy in so many words, "To reduce the birth rate to the extent necessary to stabilize the population at a level consistent with the requirement of national economy". This was the genesis of the first official National Family Planning program in the world[9]. The First Five Year Plan stated about the aspects of voluntarism by making it clear that people would be provided with advice and will be expected to go ahead on their own to plan their families. In the second half of the decade the Second Five Year Plan was declared focusing upon the increase of Family Planning Clinics from 147 to 4165.

India being one of the pioneers in Health Service Planning with a focus on Primary Health Care accepted the Bhore Committee's recommendations of establishing a well structured and comprehensive health service with a sound primary health care infrastructure. The Bhore Committee report not only provided a historical landmark in the development of the public health system but also laid down the blueprint of subsequent health planning and development in independent India[10]. Improvement in the health status of the population has been one of the major thrust areas for the social development programs of the country. This was to be achieved through improving the access to and utilization of Health, Family Welfare and Nutrition Services with special focus on under served and under privileged segment of population.

The main objectives of the First Five -Year Health Plan were; provision of water supply and sanitation; control of malaria; preventive health care; health care for mothers and children; education & training; and health education. During the first decade of plan activity, it may be justifiable claim that, training facilities had been considerably expanded; the infant and maternal mortality rate started declining. In physical terms, the first 10 years of planned development saw the establishment of 2565 primary health centers, and hospital beds had gone up to 18,500, making a bed patient ratio of 0.4 per thousand. In regard to Mother and Child Health, more than 3500 centers were started in this period.

The Planning Commissions' panel for health programs set up a committee on Population Growth and Family Planning to review the situation incorporating its key recommendations, the draft outline of the first five year plan which was released in July 1951 reported that "population policy is essential to planning" and Family Planning is a step toward "improvement in health especially of mother and children"[11] The macro effect of FP – that is a lower rate of population growth was expected to occur only "over a period of time" but it was expected to help improve health "immediately" because frequent and ill space births undermine the health of the mother.

There was a general reduction in the incidence of severe cases of anemia in areas where antenatal services were well established and a steady decrease in the infant mortality rate. During the Second Five Year Plan, Maternity and Child Welfare services became an integral part of the over-all health services in rural areas. Maternity and Child Welfare Bureaus were established in most of the States[12].

1960-70

The Sixties witnessed strengthening of mass education activities in rural areas and small towns and effective usage of traditional, cultural media like songs, drama and folk entertainment as tools to reach out to people. Strengthening of existing extension education and introduction of population education was to be as one of the strategy to bridge the gap between knowledge and adoption of family planning by couples in reproductive age groups.

Maternity and child welfare services provided by the primary health centers were supplemented by services provided by welfare extension projects and by voluntary organizations. During the Third Plan it was proposed to link up the maternity and child health services associated with the primary health units with extended facilities in referral and district hospitals. Short orientation courses were to be arranged at these hospitals for personnel engaged in maternity and child health work.

The Third Plan stated "the main appeal for family planning is based on considerations of health and welfare of the family. Family limitation or spacing of the children is necessary and desirable in order to secure better health for the mother and better care and upbringing of children. Measures directed to this end should, therefore, form part of the public health program"[13].

A sixteen-member group known as Health Survey and Planning Committee-Mudaliar Committee- was appointed to review the progress since the Bhore Committee, and assess the implementation of the First and Second Five Year Plan and make recommendations for the future. It worked through six sub-committees two services related – medical relief and public health, and two problem specific – communicable diseases and population and two, functional – education/research and stores. The Committee found that the quality of services provided by the Primary Health Centers (PHCs) were inadequate, the integration of health services as envisioned by the Committee was a non-starter and the sub-divisional and district hospitals were so weak that they could not effectively function as referral centers. It not only advised to commence the integration process and strengthen the referral centers, it also forbade establishment of new PHCs unless the existing ones were strengthened. So, the committee prioritized consolidation of institutions, rather than full coverage with minimum services to all[14]. This integrated health organization at various levels was to be operated through the Directorate of Health Services assisted by the required number of Deputy Directors for individual programs/ activities and Rural Health Centers with required number of staff.

It is important to study as to how a committee's composition can encourage it to analyze particular topic in depth. For instance both Bhore and Mudaliar paid a great deal of attention to medical education. The number of doctors in the committees and the perception of the doctor as the health team leader would have contributed to the keen interest in this topic. At the same time apart from the contextual demands of operations management posing certain larger questions, the presence of significant number of medical administrators (12 out of 16 members) and the absence of popular representatives in the Mudaliar Committee may have lead to a lesser interest in the area of community participation and popular leadership[15].

In 1961, India invited a UN Mission on Population Activities to visit the country and advise on the steps to be taken for greater acceptance of the small family norm by the population. A committee appointed by the Government of India considered the recommendations of the UN Mission. Based on the recommendations, it was decided to have the Family Planning Program as a vertical program with a separate hierarchy at the Central level, in the form of a separate Department of Family Planning, to the most peripheral level with separate workers of Family Planning. Considering the direct relationship between infant mortality and acceptance of small family norms, it was also decided to integrate the Mother and Child Health (MCH) program with Family Planning[16].

District level integration was the concern of another study group, the Eight Member, Jungalwala committee on Integration of Health Services. It was appointed in 1964 at the initiative of the Central Council of Health. Perhaps, its understanding of the administrative burdens at the state level enabled the committee to articulate the need for integration between the medical work and public health arms of the health services. Comprehensive health work was to be considered at the district level but this was not possible without requisite resources and skills.

In 1963 the report of the Director of the Family Planning (Col. B.N. Raina) for 1962-63 proposed that Family Planning should be promoted through an extension approach, with this approach specially trained auxiliary nurse midwives (now generally called female health workers) were employed by the PHCs to visit married women in their homes. The health infrastructure was to be expanded substantially even though the training facilities were inadequate to meet the needs; the population related goals were to be promoted through a large band of trainee workers who would all deliver valuable assistance with health care and childbearing to the rural population. It has been alleged that the introduction of method specific targets was a contribution of the American Management experts sent to India by the Ford Foundation, the targets were seen as essential for evaluating the performance of the program and of the personnel involved in implementing it. However, the targets also led to certain distortions that were not widely recognized for a long time. While the extension approach was supported in principle nevertheless the tyranny of targets affected the Indian Family Planning program for nearly three decades until their removal in April 1996[17].

Extension education and cafeteria approach were added to the clinical services starting from 1964. The Department of Family Planning was established in 1966. The Extension Education pattern, used by the National Program was perhaps influenced by the Gandhigram experiments in the Athoor block (1950-71). Mass vasectomy camps were launched after the successful Ernakulam camp (1972). The integration of Health and Family Planning services were tested by such pilot schemes in UP and Haryana. The Narangwal (1966-74) and Jamkhed experiments (1970-76) have shown how primary health care can be developed with the participation of the community.

As in many parts of the world in the initial stages the acceptability of the Family Planning program was assessed by questionnaire surveys of individual husbands and wives on knowledge of, and attitudes towards family planning, desire for children, and practice of family planning (Knowledge Attitude and Practices surveys). More than 200 such studies were carried out in India but very few at the national level. By and large the studies revealed that about 50% of couples approved use of family planning methods when the acceptance of family planning was much lower, questions were raised on both methodological issues and interpretation of data.

1970-80

The seventies witnessed placing of high priority to Family Planning by setting of Numerical Targets; however, the heavy reliability existed on Vasectomies. Like the previous draft of the Fourth Five Year Plan the revised draft asserted that the integration of Maternal and Child Health (MCH) with Family Planning (FP) would raise an effectiveness of the program and stated that the goal had been achieved – an assertion that seems odd given the fact that, even in 1996, the requisite coordination for integrating MCH and FP was still considered a goal to be achieved[18].

The National Programs in the field of Health and Family Planning and Nutrition had been in operation in the country for many years. In general, these programs were being run almost independently of each other by the staff recruited under each program. There was little or no coordination between the field workers or supervisory personnel of these programs. They were separate and independent functionaries. This state of affairs came into existence because the various health programs, and later on Family Planning programs were launched at different times and each was conceived to run vertically with its own staff. A question was raised in many quarters, whether the same objectives could be achieved by coordinating these programs and pooling the personnel. Accordingly the first meeting of the Executive Committee of the Central Family Planning Council held on September 20, 1972 recommended. "Steps should be taken for the integration of Medical, Public Health and Family Planning services at the peripheral level". Accordingly, the eleven member, Kartar Singh Committee was appointed in October 1972 at the initiative of the executive committee of the Central Family Planning Council[19]. The Committee on Multi-purpose Workers submitted its report in September 1973. It did consider the "integration idea" but was quite not clear, as in the case of the Jungalwalla committee, how far the attempts to strengthen the district level management were pursued by policy makers. After eliciting the views of health experts, health administrators and the community, it stated that the existing staff of the primary health centers and sub-centers cannot adequately deal with the health and family planning requirements of the population involved. The population given to each worker is too large to be adequately covered and frequently visited. The community leaders were of the view that people are not happy with the services, that so many workers were coming to their homes and making enquiries for individual programs without being in a position to tackle their health needs. On the basis of its findings the Committee recommended that, "multi-purpose workers for the delivery of Health, Family Planning and Nutritional services are both feasible and desirable."

The planner of the draft Fifth Five Year Plan confessed that many have criticized implementation, the changes suggested had been tried out but there seemed to be no improvement in the levels of performance. Considering the direct relationship between infant mortality and acceptance of small family norms, it was decided to integrate the Mother and Child Health (MCH) program with Family Planning[20]. At least in the Narangwal case, the involvement of policy makers in framing recommendations regarding the role of the health center, doctor, participation in conferences and policy analysis efforts ensured that some bridges were built between those who "study" and those who "act". The National Institute of Health Administration and Education projects (NIHAE 1971-72) to investigate the integration of health services in India and district health administration by a multi disciplinary team were also among the first such attempts in the field of general health services in India.

It was during the Fifth Five Year plan that the National Population Policy (NPP) was adopted. The NPP envisaged a series of fundamental measures including raising of the minimum age for marriage, female education, spread of population values, small family norm, strengthening of research in reproductive biology and contraception, incentives for individuals, groups and communities and permitting State Legislatures to enact legislation for compulsory sterilization.

Two hundred additional post-partum centers beyond the original targets in the draft Fifth Five Year Plan were also to be opened. Special multi-media motivation campaigns on pilot basis were to be launched in Uttar Pradesh, Andhra Pradesh, and West Bengal. Maternal and Child Health programs were to be vigorously pursued and funds for this purpose were to be made available on the basis of performance. Research and evaluation facilities were to be strengthened. Funds for completion of incomplete buildings and for construction of essential buildings for Rural Family Welfare Planning Centers were provided.

A distinguished group of social scientists and medical administrators proposed an alternative health care system. WHO/UNICEF presented a joint study on alternative approaches and later were to document alternative experiences[21]. It considered lack of a clear national health policy, poor linkage of the health system with other components of national development, lack of clear priorities and inadequate community involvement in health care as critical issues[22].

The Government of India Report (1974) of the Committee on the Status of Women in India stated "Health is both an important factor in the achievement of the status as well as an indicator of social status, particularly for women, whose health is conditioned to great extent by social attitudes. The health status of women includes their mental and social condition as affected by prevailing norms attitudes of society in addition to their biological and physiological problems. Societies definite women's roles partly according to their biological function and partly from influence the provision and use of preventive and curative health care including maternal care. The health care facilities offered by the community in the form of medical particularly maternity services for women, is significant index of the emphasis that community places on the health of its women. Some studies in the both developed and developing countries have shown a definite link between low status of women and deficiencies in the knowledge and utilization of preventive health services[23].

In the Bucharest conference (1974), India took the development approach and was credited with the coining of famous slogan "development is the best contraceptive". During this period, in formal articulation of population policies the overarching concern was fertility reduction, whereas, the other demographic variables such as mortality and migration including urbanization received much less attention. Health determinants including Reproductive Health were not in the policy agenda during this period. But two decades later in Cairo, a new policy objective was adopted that centered on the well-being of women and men and gave special emphasis to the empowerment of women[24].

However, in 1976, the population policy said that it was not possible to wait for development to take place but a frontal attack on the population problem was necessary. In 1975 after Prime Minister Mrs. Indira Gandhi had declared a period of emergency her son Sanjay began to take considerable interest in the promotion of sterilization (primarily vasectomy) to slow the rate of population growth and the political leadership in general began to show support for the use of stronger measures including compulsory sterilization to this end, and active campaign was mounted in the press and media to support legal action to sterilize the couples who already had three or more children, censorship of the press and a general climate of fear limited the expression of contrary views and created a misleading impression of consensus in favour of a coercive Population Policy. The government that came into power in the year 1977 issued a new Population Policy statement and reaffirmed the entirely voluntary nature of the Family Welfare, the terminology was changed from Family Planning to Family Welfare. It stressed upon the promotion of immunization and provision of antenatal and post-natal care for the pregnant women. It also stated that coercion of any form was not to be used, however, the employees of the state and national governments, autonomous bodies, local bodies were expected to set an example and to adopt small family norm. The revised draft of the Sixth Five Year plan tripled the outlay for Maternal & Child Health as against the outlay of Family Planning to 3.4 per cent of the plan. The Planning Commission at this time set up a working group on Population Policy. The goals proposed by this working group were incorporated into the final version of Sixth Five Year Plan, 1981-85, drafted by the Planning Commission set up by Mrs. Indira Gandhi, who had returned to power in the 1980 elections. The plan recognized the momentum of growth built into the young age distribution of the population. Accordingly the targets for sterilization were increased, however the instruments for reaching these targets remained essentially unchanged. Social pressure was to be applied against early marriages and large families, spacing methods were to be promoted among younger couples and non governmental organizations were to be involved with the family planning and population issues[25].

Increasing concern with demographic growth got translated into increasing pressure on Family Planning programs and on service delivery targets during this decade. The idea was to produce more widespread desire for smaller families, late age of marriage, girl's education, improved health services to reduce infant mortality, improved family health, alternative and enhanced roles for women, and the focus mostly was on better target achievement by service providers.

A new strategy evolved for the Fifth Five Year Plan visualized the integration of Family Planning into the general health services, particularly its Maternal and Child Health care component including Nutrition. The principle of integration was to be extended to other fields, in particular to efforts at mass motivation through the existing channels for functional literacy, worker's education, health education and social welfare. It was proposed to reorganize training programs to train multipurpose health workers to deliver integrated health care services under Minimum Needs Program. The impact of this decision to see Family Planning in its proper perspective is clearly visible in the allocation of the resources proposed for the Fifth Five Year Plan[26].

1980-90

The Eighties witnessed a massive attack on the problems of unemployment and poverty through specific programs directed towards the weaker sections of society. Special attention was focused on the education and employment of women to liberate them from dependence and insecurity, thus improving their social status, and at the same time changing of their attitudes. The adoption of National Health Policy[27] recognized the close relationship between high birth rate and high infant mortality, hence focused a high priority to the Maternal & Child Health program. Preventive, promotive and educational aspects of MCH services were given the highest priority. A close linkage of health and health-related sectors with MCH activities were developed.

The Sixth Five Year Plan stated that a vast majority of pregnant and nursing mothers, especially belonging to the low socio-economic group, live on diets, which are inadequate. The high incidence of pre-maturity, low birth weight of babies and neo-natal mortality can be attributed to poor nutritional condition among the mothers. In view of this, importance was to be given to improving the maternal nutrition status. With an increase in women's employment, the income of the household would go up thereby resulting not only in raising the nutrition and child-care in the family but also bringing down the birth rate and infant mortality rate. Further it said that Family Planning cannot be the sole responsibility of any one Department but of the Government as a whole. The areas of useful activity in each Ministry/Department in relation to Family Planning were to be identified, spelt out in precise terms, and responsibility for these activities squarely fixed on the Ministries/Departments concerned[28].

High morbidity and mortality rates among infants and mothers were generally believed to be responsible for the desire for more children and hence the aim was to bring down these rates through improvement of health and nutrition status and through various extension programs of immunization, prophylaxis, supplementary nutrition and health care services.

Limiting the growth of population was one of the main objectives of the Sixth Five Year Plan. This had to be achieved through education of the people to adopt a small family norm voluntarily, backed by appropriate programs of supplies and services. The Family Planning and Welfare programs were to be made a part of the total national effort at providing a better quality of life. The Family Welfare program was thus integrated with the Health program, especially Maternal and Child Health (MCH). The performance of the MCH program during the Sixth Five Year Plan, particularly in the field of immunization and antenatal care, was far from satisfactory. Measures for strengthening the program and increasing the child survival rate were very essential for the success of the program.

The government as a signatory to the Alma Ata Declaration on Health for All by A.D. 2000 constituted a working group to convert the HFA goals into programs. Appointed by the Planning Commission this group was to review the past plans and was to suggest measures for the Sixth Five Year Plan (1980-85), in particular, for the weaker sections. The working group asserted that health for all is achievable given the sustained will and the supporting efforts to implement the indicated task. The group tried to outline alternative objectives and strategies. Indicators were now sought in terms closer to impacts and outcomes of health programs that is reduction in mortality rate, percentage of pregnant mothers receiving ante natal care, percentage being delivered by trained birth attendants, etc[29].

The National Health Policy, 1983[30] pointed to the need of restructuring the health services- the preventive, promotive and rehabilitative aspects of health care and brought out the need for establishing comprehensive services to reach the population in the remotest areas. The programs were being implemented through the fullest involvement of the communities. It viewed health and human development as a vital component of overall socio-economic development. For the realization of the various objectives the policy indicated specified goals to be achieved by 1985, 1990 and the year 2000.

It was felt necessary that the pattern of development of the health services infrastructure in the future fully took into account the revised 20-Point Program. The said Program attributed very high priority to the promotion of Family Planning as a people's program, on a voluntary basis, acceleration of welfare programs for women and children, nutrition programs for pregnant women, nursing mothers and children, especially in the tribal, hilly and backward areas. In view of the vital importance of securing the balanced growth of the population, it was felt necessary to enunciate, separately, a National Population Policy[31].

The NHP stated that while efforts should continue at providing refresher training and orientation to the traditional birth attendants, schemes and programs should be launched to ensure that progressively all deliveries are conducted by competently trained persons so that complicated cases receive timely and expert attention, within a comprehensive program providing ante-natal, intra-natal and post-natal care.

A major change in the implementation of the Family Planning program following 1981 was the effort to promote reversible methods. The reported numbers of acceptors of IUDs, condoms, and oral contraceptives rose faster than ever before. However, there was a large extent of over reporting done (stated in the third all India survey by the Operations Research Group, Baroda, in 1989 and NFHS in 1993)[32].

The Seventh Five Year Plan stated that educating and enlightening people on the benefits of late marriage and its social enforcement was extremely necessary in order to achieve the national long-term demographic goals. Special programs and incentives oriented towards eligible couples, particularly in the younger age-groups, were needed. Inter-sectoral coordination and cooperation and the involvement of voluntary agencies in the program was felt necessary. Community Participation was essential for the voluntary acceptance of the Family Welfare program. Identification and active involvement of nongovernmental organizations and of informal leaders in the community and imparting to them the necessary training to motivate and to participate in the program were important aspects of efforts in this field[33].

As more than half of the infant mortalities are in the neo-natal period, the Maternity and Child Health program (MCH) was considerably strengthened. The MCH component of training of medical and para-medical was carefully planned and implemented. Vigorous steps will were taken to reduce maternal mortality. Since more than two-thirds of the women in the rural areas were still being attended to at childbirth by untrained Dais, the Dais training programs were initiated. A great deal of efforts were planned for special Information, Education and Communication (IEC) campaigns to remove the bias against girl children and for propagation and enforcement of the law relating to the minimum age of marriage[34].

The major thrust of MCH in accordance with the National Health Policy in the Seventh Five Year Plan was directed as follows: Recognizing the close relationship that exists between high birth rate and high infant mortality, high priority was to be given to the MCH program. Preventive, promotive and educational aspects of MCH services were given the highest priority. A close linkage of health and health-related sectors with MCH activities were developed. Health care for mothers and children was strengthened through the primary health care approach, which includes integrated, comprehensive MCH care and suitable strengthening of referral services. Increased emphasis on people's participation in MCH activities by supporting voluntary organizations, NGOs, village health committees, women's organizations, women's clubs and traditional -birth attendants was planned. **It also stated that** the health of mothers and, in particular maternal mortality, is significantly affected by induced abortions performed by unqualified persons under unhygienic conditions. Hence the Medical Termination of Pregnancy Act (MTP) (1971) was to be utilized as a legislative measure for improving maternal health through the stipulation of conditions under which pregnancies may be terminated. By the end of the Seventh Five Year Plan period, it was anticipated that MTP services would be provided at all primary health centers and in urban areas it was to be made available in all maternity homes and centers. MTP services were to be an integral part of Maternal and Child Health services and were closely linked with the same. An intensive education and publicity program making use of all available facilities was planned for improving service utilization[35].

In addition to services provided through the general health care system, the MCH program aimed at raising health consciousness among women. A comprehensive, field-based Information, Education and Communication program was developed. Women were to be organized around available economic activities to enable them to actively participate in the entire process of socio-economic development including health. Services for the health care of mothers during ante-natal, intra-natal and post-natal period were planned to be strengthened. Services of obstetricians and gynecologists were planned at the community health centers, and at sub-district and district levels.

Efforts were planned for complete integration of the organizational set-up under Health, Family Welfare and MCH programs. Financial integration towards the objective of funding all the services as a package program under a common budget head was also to be attempted by the States and the Center. The Seventh Five Year plan intended to achieve Long Term Demographic Goal by launching of Special Education Program through Mass Media. It was for the first time that special efforts were undertaken. Community participation through the use of Non-Government Organizations in Special Utilization Program was planned with the assistance from UNICEF

III. 1990 Onwards and Post ICPD Period

The nineties witnessed a sudden change in the terminologies used and the approaches determined to handle the issues related to reproductive health. The first half of the decade was spent in producing a new approach towards Reproductive Health at the national level which was to be spelt out in the draft National Population Policy (NPP), whereas the second half was fully occupied with the modifications of the programs and then complying with the international norms set in the International Conference on Population Development (ICPD), 1994.

The Eighth Five Year plan stated that the Family Planning program remained a Government program, with marginal involvement and participation from the community. Due to inadequacy of Information, Education and Communication (IEC) activities the knowledge of the community about the contraceptives, their availability, safety, etc. remained at a low level. Adoption of the small family norm and use of appropriate measures for birth control were matters of personal choice and decision. The IEC activities had to take this into account. However, till recently, the IEC activities were directed more to national issues rather than personal issues. Undoubtedly, this incongruity of perception between the people and the providers of services cost the program dearly. Inter-sectoral interaction, supported by political commitment and a popular mass movement, was to constitute the approach to strategic interventions during the plan period. A Committee of the National Development Council (NDC) on Population was constituted in February, 1992 to consider these issues and based on its report; a concrete plan of action was to be worked out[36].

The Ninth Five Year plan observed that the highest number of maternal deaths in 1995 were due to bleeding of pregnancy and puerperium which are preventable through better Reproductive Health care. Abortion, which is the second high accounted for 17.6 per cent of total maternal deaths in 1995, although abortion was legalized as early as in 1972 as a health measure through the Medical Termination of Pregnancy (MTP) Act, 1971. Despite this special sanction, illegal abortions continued to be performed by the unauthorized persons like the local quacks and untrained persons under unhygienic and unsafe conditions because of the non-availability of MTP services within the easy reach of most of the rural population. Further, about 47.5 per cent of deliveries were performed by untrained persons during 1995-96. While the Reproductive Tract Infections (RTIs) and Sexually Transmitted Infections (STIs) were already very high, cases of HIV/AIDS were also increasing amongst women. Of the total 3161 cases of AIDS reported by the end of 1996, 749 were women[37].

Improvement in the health status of women received high priority during the Ninth Five Year plan period. The erstwhile program of Maternal and Child Health services was recast as the

Child Survival and Safe Motherhood (CSSM) program and launched in 72 districts during 1992-93. The same was further expanded to cover 466 districts by the end of the Eighth Five Year plan. Under the Universal Immunization Program (UIP), the TT vaccination coverage of pregnant women increased from 40 per cent in 1985-86 to 76.4 per cent in 1996-97 and 80.93 per cent in 1997-98. These services of CSSM, as revealed by various evaluation studies, contributed significantly to the reduction of Infant Mortality Rate from 79 to 72; Crude Birth Rate from 29.2 to 27.5 and Crude Death Rate from 10 to 9.0 during 1992 to 1996. An extensive network of 2424 Community Health Centers, 22,962 Primary Health Centers and 1,36,815 village level Sub-Centers was in actual operation by 1997 to extend primary health care services including Safe Motherhood and other Family Planning services to women in rural areas[38].

After the 1991 census, the Karunakaran Committee of the National Development Council (NDC) proposed the formulation of a National Population Policy (NPP). In August 1993, an expert group headed by Dr. M.S. Swaminathan was asked to prepare a draft of NPP that would be discussed by the cabinet and then by the parliament. The draft submitted in May 1994, was subsequently circulated amongst the members of Parliament, and various agencies of the central and state governments were asked to comment. Gradually the government began to reorient the Family Planning program in light of some of the policy proposals of the Karunakaran committee, the expert group chaired by Dr. Swaminathan, and the concerns articulated in the program of action approved at the ICPD 1994[39].

Prevention and control of the misuse of medical technologies for commercial purposes was taken up on a priority basis as the incidence of female foeticide has been on an increase due to misuse of the medical technology of Amniocentesis for sex determination, which is generally followed by illegal and harmful practices of female foeticide. Action in this direction included effective enforcement of the Pre-Natal Diagnostic Techniques (PNDT) (Regulation and Prevention of Misuse) Act, 1994 with stringent measures of punishment of both the parties. Efforts were also to be made to create an enabling environment for women to exercise their reproductive rights and choices freely, so as to contain the population growth[40].

After being a signatory to the ICPD, India immediately declared about the removal of targets of the existing Family Planning program, however the actual Reproductive and Child Health (RCH) program as per the ICPD was launched in India in 1997. The program was to be implemented in all states as per the guidelines stated by the central government. The guidelines were formulated in accordance with the Program of Action (POA) of the ICPD. Under RCH care, steps for prevention and treatment of gynecological problems including infertility, menstrual disorders, screening and treatment of cancers especially that of breast and uterine cervix etc. were planned to be taken up. Also, the traditional health care, especially practiced by women, was encouraged through programs of Indian Systems of Medicine. Gender-sensitive initiatives that address the sexually transmitted infections/diseases (STDs), HIV/AIDS and other sexual and reproductive health issues, were to be attended to on a priority basis.

The health education material, being brought out as part of IEC material for family planning, was being made gender sensitive for both men and women. Special efforts were made to disseminate information to women, especially in rural and tribal areas on the available Reproductive Health services. Efforts to promote participation of men in planned parenthood, in increasing acceptance of vasectomy and active co-operation of men in STD/ RTI Prevention Control, was to receive priority attention[41]. The guidelines formulated by Government of India stated that the importance of IEC activity cannot be overstated for demystifying the RCH and population issues among public and in advocacy role. Imaginatively produced programs have a very strong persuasive effect. Therefore, the Department of Family Welfare has been implementing a large IEC program under which extensive use is being made of Doordarshan, All India Radio, Directorate of Advertising and Visual Publicity, Directorate of Field publicity, Song and Drama division and Films Division under the Ministry of Information and Broadcasting. In addition, Mahila Swasthya Sanghs, sensitization of opinion leaders, health awareness units in Nehru Yuva Kendras are being supported[42].

After Cairo, policy decision-making gave precedence to individual Reproductive Health needs over the previous concern with reducing family size norms, quality of care was to have priority over long-range objectives and targets of demography and services were to be integrated. In this process Family Planning became just one component among an array of service options aiming at improving women's health and well being. Men were for the first time recognized as actors in family formation and decision making as well as potential vectors in the transmission of disease to their partners and thus were also be targeted by services. In short, the scope of the Reproductive Health approach, as laid out in the POA was not only revolutionary in intent but also formidable in terms of the effort it was to take to make it viable and attainable. An important component of the task ahead was to generate and commit resources needed both professional and financial[43].

By attempting to estimate the long-term cost of implementing the Reproductive Health and Family Planning components of the POA, Cairo was the first UN conference to link policy to implementation. The initial results of this estimation is some what unsatisfactory, largely because, unlike the cost of Family Planning programs which is reasonably well known, data on which to base estimate of implementing Reproductive Health services are scarce. The proposed distribution of cost between donor and recipient countries, one third to be provided by donors and two third by recipient countries-compared to the estimated present division of approximately five per cent from external assistance and private sources and seventy five per cent from recipient governments-was thought to be out of reach by both sides. The development issues raised in the Cairo document deserved far greater attention than the international community has given them in recent decades. In essence, they dealt with the distribution of wealth and power and thus had a critical bearing on some of the most troubling questions of our time, mainly the increasing poverty and indebtedness of many developing countries. Significantly, the change of direction, which paid less heed to demographic and development objectives than to women's issues, was brought about indirectly by the high level of NGO participation in the Cairo process. The inclusion of NGOs in the preparatory process fostered a new, sharper discourse and disrupted the complaisance of the rigid bureaucratic political structures that are characteristic of many developing countries.

Internationally, the issues of democratic representation and accountability were made more complex by the fact that donor governments and foundations were instrumental in facilitating and the funding the participation of a significant number of NGOs from developing countries. While this is understandable and may have been unavoidable given the limited financial resources of many third world countries and NGOs, the question of accountability and representative ness remain. Not withstanding these problems, it is clearly desirable to include some kind of popular or civic participation in the policymaking process at UN conferences. The method used to achieve this objective at Cairo was somewhat deficient, but the issue is one that deserves continued attention[44].

It is evident that in the field of social policy UN conferences have become an institutionalized part of international relations. As a means of policy formulation, global conferences serve an important function in permitting the expression of views that might not otherwise be aired, and in widening the circle of decision makers. In this regard the Cairo conference may have exceeded expectations. It delivered very effectively a number of messages about the status and aspirations of women, the strengths and limits of papal power, the vitality of NGOs, and the unequal distribution of power and influence in the world. At the same time, it demonstrated weaknesses that may be endemic in the UN system of global meetings. Inevitably, given the structure and conventions of the United Nations, these large global meetings produce an unwieldy, excessively comprehensive, and indigestible set of recommendations that bind no one. Ironically, some of the hard prioritizing that UN conference are unable to accomplish is, in the case of Cairo, taking place as governments, UNFPA, donors, and some NGOs struggle over how to implement the POA under severe resource constraints.[45].

RCH approach was built upon the participatory planning approach that was initiated in 1996-97. The participatory planning approach was intended to identify RCH needs of the communities and clients and the Target Free Approach manual is an instrument to assist this process. Target Free manual, which was renamed as Community Needs Assessment Manual was revised in order to simplify the messages and contents and is available to all districts for distribution among all health facilities and workers. On the basis of community needs assessed by the health workers, Sub-centre Action Plan were to be prepared annually. This process involves discussion and approval of supervisor of the health worker (LHV/MO). Similarly PHC Action Plan incorporates the Sub-centre Action Plan prepared under the supervision of the next supervisory officer. The PHC plans form an integral part of the District plan, which is formulated on annual basis. Availability of the Annual District Plan is considered to be one of the performance indicator[46].

One of the policy evaluation study noted that the transition from a centrally controlled and top-down program to a program with more state control and bottom-up planning required an adjustment period before it can be fully implemented and demonstrate a level of success. India's basic package of essential RCH services is supposed to be delivered through integrated services. In many ways, the existing service delivery infrastructure has become increasingly integrated. In 1965, Family planning was integrated with MCH and Nutrition services. In 1992, the Child Survival and Safe Motherhood (CSSM) program integrated key child survival interventions with safe motherhood and Family Planning activities. The RCH Project includes RTIs, STDs and strengthening of abortion as well as referral services. Despite the high level of integration, vertical programs within the MOHFW still exist. As the primary STD/AIDS program, National AIDS Control Organization has a separate delivery system of STD clinics[47].

One of the ICPD's most significant contributions has been the elimination of contraceptive method-specific targets, which is especially important for female sterilization procedures. India has defined a basic package of essential RCH services that includes planning with sterilization services, social marketing, distribution of oral contraceptives and condoms, provision of intrauterine devices (IUDs), maternity care, including prenatal, delivery and postpartum services, child survival, breastfeeding, nutrition, immunization, growth monitoring, acute respiratory infection detection and management, immunization, A-Vitamin supplementation, diarrhea management, Prevention and management of RTIs/STDs, including detection by using the syndromic approach and antenatal screening for syphilis[48].

The POA which was agreed to by 180 countries represented at the ICPD reaffirmed the importance of slowing population growth for social and economic development but it also called for a significant shift in strategies to achieve this goal. Rather than continuing a supply side and quantitative approach to achieve demographic targets the ICPD endorsed a client driven approach to meet Reproductive Health needs of individual women men and their families. It emphasized the interrelationships between population, human rights and sustainable development, and stressed the importance of advancing gender equality, equity and the empowerment of women. It emphasized women's ability to control their own fertility. It promoted women's involvement in the planning, management, implementation, and evaluation of Reproductive Health programs and emphasized the role of men as active partners in Family Planning and family lives. It recommended the primary healthcare systems in all countries to provide a range of Reproductive Health information and services including but not limited to Family Planning.

The Government of India launched an innovative Reproductive and Child Health program in October 1997, shifting from a bureaucratic, target-driven program to a client-centered, gender-sensitive program focused on delivering high-quality care. This change reflects consensus—reached at the 1994 International Conference on Population and Development—that greater social equity and reduced population growth would result from such policies[49].

In order to implement the RCH program with a target free approach, a number of drawbacks related to the target based approach were assessed immediately. One of the drawbacks of the top down target approach was that the quality of service became secondary and did not receive due attention. If the targets for sterilization were to be achieved but the complications were at a high rate because the quality of service was compromised while selecting and dealing with cases for sterilization, the net result would be negative. Similarly in the case of IUD, if the discontinuation rate was very high because in the attempt to fulfill targets for the number of IUD insertions, the quality of care was compromised, especially while screening women for pre-existing RTI and STI before IUD insertion, the acceptability of the IUD program received a serious set back. Another disadvantage that was observed with the top down target approach was that people were tempted to resort to false reporting to claim laurels for having fulfilled the targets. According to the National Family Health Survey conducted in 1992-93, the percentage of contraceptive acceptance was less than those indicated by the statistics provided by the districts and state Governments. It was also noted that the state, which had reported a high acceptance rate for sterilization had not achieved corresponding reduction in the birth rate[50].

The RCH program incorporated the components of the Child Survival and Safe Motherhood program and further included two additional components- one relating to sexually transmitted diseases (STD) and the other relating to reproductive tract infection (RTI). A study on policy analysis of India after the declaration of implementing RCH stated that "In real terms, recurrent expenditures for health and family welfare declined from 1991 to 1994. To implement the Reproductive Health approach fully, India will have to make a strong financial commitment to increasing program funding. With structural adjustment measures underway, it seems unlikely that the Indian government-with its mixed support for Reproductive Health – will be able to meet its financing challenge on its own. Donors are increasing their aid to the program, and some experts expect donor funds to continue to increase and play a larger role in the program in the future[51].

It is felt that the Reproductive Health programs should aim to reduce the burden of unplanned and unwanted childbearing and related morbidity and mortality[52]. The challenges faced by the program are enormous. Although reproductive health policy has been articulated, it will be several years before judgments can be made on the success of the initiative. Yet, concrete steps to create more informed choice, meet individuals needs, improve quality, and develop a participatory process all seem to be leading the program in the appropriate direction.

The National Population Policy 2000 and Reproductive Health

Public Health Policy development has a long history in India, which launched its NFP program in 1952. India has been a leader in calling for broad integrated approaches to population as it did during the first United Nations World Population Conference, held in Bucharest in 1974. India continues to affirm its commitment to slowing population growth a priority area in the Eighth Five Year plan, and in its statement to the ICPD, 1994. Despite many successes including a doubling in contraceptive prevalence from around 20% in the early seventies to more than 40% by the early 1990s, the Family Welfare program continues to suffer from longstanding problems of implementation many of which have their roots in policy. These problems have been addressed in the "Action plan for revamping the Family Welfare program in India" which was drawn up by the MOHFW in 1992[53]. In 1952 India was the first country in the world to launch a National Program emphasizing Family Planning. After 1952, sharp decline in death rates were however not accompanied by a similar drop in birth rates. The National Health Policy, 1983 stated that replacement level of total fertility rate (TFR) should be achieved by the year 2000. Though the NPP states that stabilizing population is an essential requirement for promoting sustainable development with more equitable distribution, it however focuses on the function of making Reproductive Health care accessible and affordable for all, as of increasing the provision and out reach of primary and secondary education extending basic amenities including sanitation, safe drinking water and housing, besides empowering women and enhancing their employment opportunities, and providing transport and communication.

The NPP 2000[54] provides a policy framework for advancing goals and prioritizing strategies during the next decade to meet the Reproductive and Child Health needs of the people of India, and to achieve net replacement level (TFR) by 2010. It is based upon the need to simultaneously address issues of child survival, maternal health, and contraception, while increasing out reach and coverage of a comprehensive package of RCH services by government, industry and the voluntary non-government sector, working in partnership.

Programs for safe motherhood, Universal Immunization, Child Survival and Oral Re-hydration, have been combined into an integrated RCH Program, Which also includes promoting management of STIs and RTIs. Further emphasis is laid on the IEC of Family Welfare messages, to be strengthened and their outreach widened, with locally relevant, and locally comprehensible media.

REFERENCES

1. United Nations, "*Program of Action-International Conference on Population and Development*", (Cairo, 1994).
2. K. Srinivasan, *Regulating Reproduction in India's Population – Efforts, Results and Recommendations*, New Delhi, Sage Publications. p. 17.
3. *Ibid.*, p. 20.
4. Saumya Panda, *Evolution of India's Health Policy 1947 – 2001 An Appraisal*, (Indian Academy of Social Sciences, Allahabad, 2002). p. 10.
5. Subhash Kashyap, *National Policy Studies*, (The Lok Sabha Secretariat, New Delhi, India,Tata McGraw-Hill Publishing Company Limited, 1990), p. 378.
6. K. Srinivasan, n. 2, p. 23.
7. Subhash Kashyap, n. 5 p. 378.
8. Subhash Kashyap, n. 5, p. 379.
9. K. Srinivasan, n. 2, p. 29.
10. Government of India, *Ninth Five Year Plan*, Vol. 2.,– Health, (New Delhi, Planning Commission, 1997) Col. 3.4.1.
11. Government of India, Planning Commission, *Document 16*, (New Delhi, 1951), p. 206, 207.
12. Government of India, *Third Five Year Plan*, (New Delhi, Planning Commission 1961).
13. *Ibid.*
14. Saumya Panda, n. 4, p. 12.
15. R.S. Ganpathy, S.R. Ganesh, Rushikesh Maru, Samuel Paul, Ram Mohan Rao, *Public Policy and Policy Analysis in India*, (New Delhi, India, Sage Publications, 1985), p 93.
16. Subhash Kashyap, n. 5, p. 383.
17. Anrudh Jain, *Do Population Policies Matter? — Fertility and Policies in Egypt, India, Kenya and Mexico*, (New York, Population Council, 1998), p. 62-63.
18. Anrudh Jain, n. 17, p. 66-67.
19. R.S. Ganpathy et.al., n. 15, p. 95.
20. Subhash Kashyap, n. 5, p. 383.
21. R.S. Ganpathy et.al., n.15, p. 98.
22. R.S. Ganpathy et al, n.15, p. 98.
23. Government of India, *Towards Equality* (Report of the Committee on the Status of Women in India, New Delhi, 1974), p. 310.

24. Shepard Forman and Romita Ghosh, *Promoting Reproductive Health-Investing in Health for Development*, (London, Lynne Rienner Publishers, 2000), p. 281.
25. Anrudh Jain, n. 17, p. 72-73.
26. *Towards Equality* n. 25, p. 325.
27. Subhash Kashyap, n. 5, pp. 387-391.
28. Government of India, *Sixth Five Year Plan*, (New Delhi, Planning Commission1980).
29. R.S. Ganpathy et al, n. 15, p. 99.
30. Subhash Kashyap, n. 5, pp. 404-418.
31. Subhash Kashyap, n. 5, p. 405.
32. Anrudh Jain, n.17, p. 72-73.
33. Government of India, *Seventh Five Year Plan*, (New Delhi, Planning Commission 1985), Col. 11.75
34. *Ibid.*, Col. 11.78.
35. Government of India, *Seventh Five Year Plan*, (New Delhi, Planning Commission 1985).
36. Government of India, *Eighth Five Year Plan*, (New Delhi, Planning Commission 1992), Col. 12.4.11, 12.5.2.
37. Government of India, *Ninth Five Year Plan*, (New Delhi, Planning Commission 1997), Col. 3.8.9.
38. *Ibid.*, Col. 3.8.61.
39. Anrudh Jain, n.17, p. 74.
40. Government of India, *Ninth Five Year Plan*, (New Delhi, Planning Commission 1997), Col. 3.8.34.
41. *Ibid.*, Col.3.8.35.
42. Government of India, *Reproductive and Child Health Programme*, (New Delhi, India Ministry of Health and Family Welfare, Govt. of India, 1997), p. 31.
43. Shepard Forman and Romita Ghosh, n. 26, p. 282.
44. C. Alison McIntosh, Jason L. Finkle, "The Cairo Conference on Population and Development: A new Paradigm?", *Population and Development Review*, Vol. 21, No. 2, June 1995. p. 250.
45. *Ibid.*, p. 252.
46. *Reproductive and Child Health Program*, n. 44, p. 39-40.

47. Karen Hardee, Kokila Agarwal, Nancy Luke, Ellen Wilson, Margaret Pendzich, Marguerite Farrell, Harry Cross, *Post Cairo Reproductive Health Policies and Programs: A Comparative Study of Eight Countries*, (Washington DC, USAID, 1998), p. 25.

48. *Ibid.*, p. 7.

49. Saroj Pachauri, *Defining a Reproductive Health Package for India: A Proposed Framework, South and East Asia* – (Regional Working Papers, New Delhi, The Population Council, 1995).

50. Government of India, *Manual on Community Needs Assessment Approach in Family Welfare Program*, (New Delhi, India, Ministry of Health and Family Welfare, Government of India, 1998), p. 10-15.

51. Karen Hardee et al, n.48, 1998, p 31.

52. Saroj Pachauri, n. 51, p 7.

53. Anthony Measham and Richard Heaver, *Supplement to India's Family Welfare Program-Moving to Reproductive and Child Health Approach*, Washington, The World Bank, 1996, p. 13.

54. Government of India, *National Population Policy*, (Ministry of Health and Family Welfare, New Delhi, 2000).

4

Communication Strategies in Reproductive Health

Introduction

This Chapter focuses upon the policies related to Reproductive Health in general and Health Education and Communication Strategies applied in the field of Reproductive Health in particular.

I. Communication Campaigns in India

Health Education is not a new concept in India. Traditionally Health Education/Information was propagated through face-to-face communication; but formalized/institutional structures did not exist. The principles of health were interwoven with local cultural and religious practices.

The aim of Health Education is best summarized earliest in the report of the first expert committee on Health Education that met in Geneva in 1953: "The aim of Health Education is to help people to achieve health by their own actions and efforts. Health Education begins, therefore, with the interest of people in improving their conditions of living and aims at developing a sense of responsibility for their own health betterment as individuals, and as members of families, communities and governments. Health is but one of the elements in the general welfare of people, and Health Education is only one of the factors in improving health and social conditions. It is, however, an indispensable factor and therefore should be integrated with the other social, economic, health and educational efforts.[1]"

Though there has always been a confusion regarding the usage of terminology related to Health Education and Health Communication, the term Information, Education and Communication or IEC was adopted as a compromise to avoid the need for consensus on any one of the three terms, each of which has different connotations and academic origins. Over the last twenty-five years however, the term "Communication" has gradually become the general concept that encompasses the other two[2].

In the era when Reproductive Health as a terminology had not evolved, communication was being linked to only the Family Welfare programs, which supposedly involved the elements of Reproductive Health also. By the early seventies, general knowledge of Family Planning had already begun reaching out to people, at this time two major reviews of family planning communication were published. They provided a benchmark to measure both the status of these early programs and progress. In 1971, Wilbur Schramm's review, "Communication in Family Planning", was published by the Population Council, and in 1973 Everett Rogers' ground breaking "Communication Strategies for Family Planning" appeared. Both of these expert reviews covered the experience of population programs in 11 countries and communication inputs in 20 national programs; out of these only 5 countries: India, Iran, Kenya, South Korea and Taiwan had official Family Planning policies[3].

In last five decades India has had several communication campaigns, producing mixed results. While looking at these campaigns it is equally important to understand the scientific approach required to be adopted in successful communication campaigns. With the ultimate aim being that of **behaviour change**, the various steps involved are:

- Firstly, **Knowledge** – leading to understanding of the concept by the client;
- Secondly, **Approval** – leading to favourable response to the information gained;
- Thirdly, **Intention** – leading to recognition of the idea;
- Fourthly, **Practice** – leading to actual use of the information;
- Lastly, **Advocacy** – leading to advocating and transfer of the same knowledge to others.

All the abovementioned five steps lead to behaviour change in people and hence considering these steps is very necessary in actually analyzing the results of any communication campaign undertaken.

Communication being represented by different terminologies has been a part of all the policy statements emerging in India from time to time. The National Health Policy-1983 stated that the recommended efforts, on various fronts, would bear only marginal results unless nation-wide Health Education programs, backed by appropriate Communication Strategies are launched to provide health information in easily understandable form, to motivate the development of an attitude for healthy living. The Public Health Education programs should be supplemented by Health, Nutrition and Population Education programs in all educational institutions. Simultaneously, efforts would require to be made to promote universal education, specially adult and family education, without which the various efforts to organize preventive and promotive health activities, Family Planning and improved Maternal and Child Health cannot bear fruit[4].

The National Population Policy 2000 states that Information, Education and Communication (IEC) of Family Welfare messages must be clear, focused and disseminated everywhere, including to the remote corners of the country and in local dialects. This will ensure that the messages are effectively conveyed. These need to be strengthened and their outreach widened, with locally relevant and locally comprehensible media and messages[5].

With regards to the Communication Strategies the Program of Action adopted at the ICPD, Cairo, 1994 spells out that "Effective Information, Education and Communication are prerequisites for sustainable human development and pave the way for attitudinal and behavioural change. Indeed, this begins with the recognition that decisions must be made freely, responsibly, and in informed manner. On the number and spacing of children and in all other aspects of daily life, including sexual and reproductive behaviour"[6].

The Government of India Commission on the Status of Women (1974) stated that, in any country, women who are half of the total population are often half the audience. The success or failure of the development plans, in education, in Family Planning, community development, health and nutrition depends upon involvement and participation of the women. Investigation showed that compared to men, women are underprivileged in many ways and suffer from serious disabilities. Since formal education is costly and a long term process, it is essential to harness mass media for eradication of illiteracy and to speed up the spread of basic education among women and girls. The National Council for Women's Education emphasized the potential significance of the mass media to generate public opinion in rural areas in favour of girls' education. Incidental studies on the impact of the mass media indicated, however, that women's exposure to media was often very inadequate, and unsatisfactory. It appears that the mass media had not been effective instrument to inform and prepare women to play their new role in society. The committee's investigations indicated a general lack of the awareness about the rights, problems, opportunities and responsibilities among both men and women[7].

In the discussion of the high rates of masculinity of India's population, incidence of disproportionately high rates of female mortality in regions with depressed sex ratio has been cited. The reasons for this excess mortality are far from clear. Two culturally related factors — discrimination in nutrition and access to health care — have been proposed by a number of investigators[8].

The deficiencies in the implementation of various abovementioned policies partly reflect India's democratic structure and the plurality of its population rather than inadequate recognition of the action that need to be taken. India's earliest Population Policy like the policies in many other countries is not articulated in a single document nevertheless the various document relating to India's Five Year plans for social and economic development contain an excellent record of the milestones and the factors guiding various decisions concerning the countries Population Policy. It is often argued that population policies in developing country reflect, to a large extent, pressure from industrialized countries rather than an indigenous consensus in favour of limiting population growth. Even if this assertion is true India is an exception as evidenced by the country's history both before and after it achieved independence from Great

Britain in 1947. The concern about the fertility level (the no. of children born to Indian women) and about the rate of population growth was not enforced on India from abroad, the country's leaders had been exposed to the development in western countries and did not want India to lag behind.

The demographic and health profile of the country is not uniform; the examination of the state wide data regarding behaviour of the important demographic and health indicators shows very clearly that any operational strategy to be successful will have to be based on disaggregated approach. The four states of Bihar, MP, Rajasthan and UP which constitute about 40% of the country's population have IMR and MMR levels distinctly higher than the national average. These are also the states where female age at marriage, female literacy and share of women in agricultural employments are distinctly lower than the national average unless special efforts are made to bring up the profile and performance of these states in regard to Health and Family Welfare. It would be well nigh impossible to accelerate the achievement of demographic and family welfare goals at the national level. Special area development projects have been already been launched in these states with the help of world bank, UNFPA and other funding agencies, the pace of the implementation of these projects primarily designed to strengthen the infrastructure and to improve the training of their staff is being speeded up with due attention to quality of implementation[9].

A number of socio economic and cultural factors have enforced the country to take up initiatives in communication campaigns with the following issues in mind. The cultural norms that particularly affect women's health are attitudes to marriage and age of marriage, the value attached to the fertility and sex of the child, the pattern of family organization and the ideal role demanded of the women by social conventions. They determine her place within family, the degree of her access to medical care, education, nutrition and other accessories of the health. The young girls as they grow up are thought subservience and self-effacement. The process, therefore, starts at an early age and has very adverse consequences on women's health particularly at the time of pregnancy and childbirth.

From their childhood, girls are taught to be uncomplaining and to maintain strict secrecy about their physical troubles. With menstruation, taboos are enforced and restrictions are placed on their movements. They are unable to discuss their health problems, if any, or even visit the doctor. Later as a mother, with children depending on her for care and attention, the women has tendency to carry on until ailment overtakes her. Reluctance to visit a doctor, particularly a male doctor, arises out of these restrictions imposed on women from the beginning. Such social attitudes, therefore, lead to general neglect of women's health and in view of their childbearing role; they are greatest sufferers as compared to men.

The specific factors that have been identified by various studies are firstly pregnancy wastages, caused by abortion and still births. The incidence of the phenomenon has remained constant over the period 1957-68, a period, which witnessed intensification of Family Planning activity. In fact there was even an increase in actual numbers. Such fetal wastage prevails more in low-income groups. One study reported that pregnancy wastage of malnourished mother was 30% as late as in 1972. Still-births were reported as constituting 11 per 1000 live births. Much of this pregnancy loose and prenatal mortality is caused by premature births and malnutrition. Perinatal mortality and still births results from premature births, itself a consequence of maternal malnutrition, particularly iron deficiency during pregnancy. Hemoglobin estimations carried out on about 5000 pregnant women in different parts of country showed that 30% of them were anemic, i.e. they have hemoglobin level below 10%. Frequency of pregnancies caused protein malnutrition of the mothers. As it is majority of Indian women are victims of malnutrition. 10-20% of maternal deaths are known to be due to nutritional anemia[10].

The Dharwar Surveys on the attitudes towards family planning undertaken by the Dharwar Demographic Research Centre in 1962 and 1969 indicated that educational level was the most important factor associated with awareness about Family Planning. While all the major surveys found a positive relationship between education and knowledge, acceptance and practice of family planning; most of them have revealed the other associational factors, which influenced this relationship. Education is generally associated with one or more of the following: rise in the age of marriage; diversification of consumption pattern of people involving both material and non material aspects which can lead to a decline in the psychic utility generated by the birth of children; urbanization; possible increase in work force participation of women; higher socioeconomic status of the couple; higher mobility; higher exposure to mass media and more diversified knowledge of Family Planning methods.[11]

The Constitution (seventy-ninth Amendment) Bill 1992, talked about radio being used as a powerful medium for disseminating the message condemning female feticide, and the strict punishment that will be meted out to anybody violating the law. Several of All India Radio programmes are broadcasting spots, group discussions, talks and panel discussions on PNDT Act in different languages. Two spots are being telecast once a week on the national network and a film "NIRANKUSH" is being telecast on the Punjabi channel in respect of the PNDT Act. NFDC has been asked to produce a small film on female feticide. A film "ATMAJA" produced by Plan International India on female foeticide is also being telecast on national channel of Doordarshan[12].

The NPP states that the Information Education and Communication (IEC) component of the National Family Welfare Programs aims to generate demand for the range of Family Welfare and Reproductive and Child Health Services available for healthy living. The Department of Family Welfare started the process of defining a holistic and yet flexible strategy for communication of the country's RCH program. Starting with a National Workshop in January 1999, followed by three regional workshops in the summer of 1999 and a series of deliberations, the National Communication Strategy was adopted through a National Workshop in October 2000. The strategy lays down the goal and suggests operational framework for communication at Central, States and District levels. It also identifies the major behavior change objectives that the communication managers have to address and achieve along with the barriers and opportunities that are in place. A crucial feature of the new strategy is the recognition that, increasingly, IEC work will have to be taken over by the States, Districts and community leaders.

The central government will continue to play the lead role in national mass media campaign and multi-media campaigns like the pulse polio immunization. While the States and districts also need to access local radio, TV and the print media, local specific IEC work through leaflets, posters, traditional entertainment methods, banners, hoardings etc. will be the exclusive responsibility of the district and community levels.

As part of the new strategy to utilize the services of eminent filmmakers, the Department of Family Welfare assigned a few full length feature films to the eminent directors such as Shri Amol Palekar, Shri Shyam Benegal, Ms. Kalpana Lazmi, Shri K. Rangaraj and Shri Sushant Mishra for feature films on Reproductive Health issues. Some of the films produced are Kalpana Lazmis film "Daman" on domestic violence, "Kal Ka Aadmi" by Amol Palekar a biographical film on Raghunath. D. Karve, the man who promoted family welfare program in the early years of the 20th century[13].

The earlier experience of the Ministry of Health and Family Welfare (MOHFW) and the Ministry of Information and Broadcasting in successfully increasing integration suggests another opportunity for implementing the Reproductive Health approach. Previously, the Ministry reported to the MOHFW when designing special campaigns on such topics as immunization, the girl-child, unequal access to food, and contraception. But now, according to one study, the two ministries do not communicate with each other. The study also reflects that the firstly, government is approaching the Reproductive Health issues very simplistically and trying to do things too fast. Secondly, complicated factors of Reproductive Health like Reproductive Tract Infections (RTIs) are a very difficult area to work in and that there is no standardization of drugs, there exists difficulty in RTI screening, until some quick and simple tests become available, and that the syndromic approach has not been transferred to the grassroots level[14].

A strategic campaign that began in Uttar Pradesh showed some of the new directions being pursued. With a population of 165 million people, Uttar Pradesh is the largest state in India, equivalent in population size to the fifth largest country in the world. Despite a total fertility rate (TFR) of 5.4 children per woman, modern contraceptive method use reached only 18.5 per cent. To address the situation, the United States Agency for International Development (USAID) and the Government of India established the Innovations in Family Planning Services project in 1992. The goal of the project is to reduce TFR to less than 4.0 and increase the modern contraceptive prevalence rate to 35 per cent by 2004.

Formative communication strategy research identified the lack of open discussion about family planning and modern methods as a key inhibitor among all intended audiences. In fact, additional research indicated that only 32 per cent of rural couples ever discussed family planning and 46 per cent of family planning decisions were made by someone other than the wife[15]. A professional advertising agency was hired which developed a comprehensive interpersonal and mass media campaign centered around the slogan "Come Let's Talk". This campaign theme is illustrated by the *tota* and *mynah* birds, well recognized in India as male and female mythical characters that are known for their talkative nature. Their benefit-focused messages are contained in entertaining poetry, riddles and banter intended to stimulate dialogue between couples, their in-laws, friends and relatives as well as policy makers and service providers, all in a non-threatening, non-controversial but action-oriented way. These mnemonic characters have been featured in a mass media campaign on television and radio, in the press and wall paintings, as well as incorporated into more than 600 entertainment-education performances of folk media, including puppet shows, street theatre, ballad songs and traditional singing groups. The entertainment-education approach was also used to link the campaign to service delivery through a massive counseling training program which oriented more than 9,000 field staff through health *melas* (fairs or festivals) and interactive workshops[16]. This client-centered campaign is helping to reposition Family Planning in India from a government quota program to a "people's programme", with strategic communication offering better informed families something positive to talk about.

Nevertheless, when Wilbur Schramm and Everett Rogers reviewed the state of Family Planning Communication Programs in the early 1970s, they highlighted a number of important weaknesses. These included; minimal coherent communication planning or strategic design to define and achieve specific goals; a failure of communication campaigns using single or multimedia to integrate their messages with existing service delivery programs on the assumption that awareness would automatically lead to action; "one-size-fits-all" messages disseminated to the general public rather than specific appeals to different segments of the audience; limited pre-testing of messages with intended audiences; little application of scientific theories of behaviour change in relation to communication in developing messages and activities; and lack of indicators and other evaluation tools to determine the impact of any communication interventions[17].

II. Constitutional Provisions

The country's concern in safeguarding the rights and privileges of women found its best expression in the Constitution of India. While Article 14 confers equal rights and opportunities on men and women in the political, economic and social spheres, Article 15 prohibits discrimination against any citizen on the grounds of sex, religion, race, caste etc. Article 15(3) empowers the state to make affirmative discrimination in favour of women. Similarly, Article 16 provides for equality of opportunities in the matter of public appointments for all citizens; Article 39 stipulates that the state shall direct its policy towards providing men and women equally the right to means of livelihood and equal pay for equal work; Article 42 directs the state to make provisions for ensuring just and humane conditions of work and maternity relief; and article 51(A)(e) imposes a fundamental duty on every citizen to renounce practices derogatory to the dignity of women. To make this de jure equality into a de-facto one, many policies and programs were put into action from time to time, besides enacting/ enforcing special legislations in favour of women.

Women as an independent target group account for 495.74 million and represent 48.3 per cent of country's total population, as per 2001 Census. Women in the reproductive age group 15-44 years numbering 233.72 million (47.1 per cent) need special care and attention because of their reproductive needs[18].

Development of women has been receiving attention of the government right from the very First Five Year plan. But, the same has been treated as a subject of 'welfare' and clubbed together with the welfare of the disadvantaged groups like destitute, disabled and aged. The Central Social Welfare Board (CSWB), set up in 1953, acts as an apex body at national level to promote voluntary action at various levels, especially at the grassroots, to take up welfare related activities for women and children. The Second to Fifth Five Year Plans continued to reflect the very same welfare approach, besides giving priority to women's education, and launching measures to improve maternal and child health services, supplementary feeding for children and expectant and nursing mothers.

III. The Five-Year Plans

Policy statements have been made in each Five-Year plan. As is relevant for the study, it is necessary to track down the major decisions and changes taking place in the declarations and statements of the Five Year plans related to two aspects one being that of Health in general and Reproductive Health in particular, the second being that of Health Education.

The **First Five Year Plan** in its chapter 32 stated "Health involves primarily the application of medical science for the benefit of the individual and of society. But many other factors, social, economic and educational have an intimate bearing on the health of the community. Health is thus a vital part of a concurrent and integrated program of development of all aspects of community life"[19]. It further asserted that the present low state of Public Health is reflected in the wide prevalence of disease and the high rate of mortality in the community as a whole and in particular among vulnerable groups such as children and women in their reproductive age period. Maternity and Child Health was a service that was kept in the forefront in the planning of health programs. The protection of the health of the expectant mother and her child was considered to be of utmost importance for building a sound and healthy nation.

With regards to Health Education it declared that to be effective, Health Education should be addressed to the different sections of the public in a manner suitable to each. Women and children constitute the most important section, not only all available modern methods of publicity were to be adopted but, that they should be as attractive as possible and intelligible to the large section, those are not literate. Audio-visual aids, the radio, the cinema, and the press were to be extensively utilized. Television would come into use in due course. Gramophone records, cinema films, film strips, lantern slides, picture posters, leaflets, book marks and picture cards were to be produced and spread widely to the public in any attempt at effective publicity. The material prepared for imparting health knowledge to the people was to draw upon all available sources, including the traditional practices and Ayurvedic texts[20].

It further reiterated that to organize this work, it is essential to have health publicity bureaus in the Centre as well as the States. Family limitation or spacing of the children is necessary and desirable in order to secure better health for the mother and better care and upbringing of children. Measures directed to this end, therefore, formed part of the Public Health program.

The **Second Five Year Plan** stressed upon the provision of about Rs. 3 crores by the state for the setting up of about 2,100 Maternity and Child Health Centers. These centers were to be integrated with the primary health unit services. The need for proper training of medical and ancillary personnel to be employed in Maternal and Child Health programs was recognized and the plan made the necessary provision. It reiterated that the primary object of Health Education is to help the people to achieve health by their own action and efforts[21].

As per the **Third Five Year Plan** in its widest sense Health Education is the very foundation of a successful Public Health program. To implement the program of health education, the Central Health Bureau was established in 1956 in the Directorate General of Health Services and several States had also set up such Bureaus. Among the most important aspects of Health Education were personal hygiene, environmental sanitation, prevention of communicable diseases, nutrition, physical exercise, marriage guidance, pre-natal and post-natal care, maternity and child health, etc. Maternity and Child Welfare Bureaus were established in most of the States[22].

The **Fourth Five Year Plan** provided with the details of implementation mechanisms. It laid down the importance of making annual plans, and the planning at state and district level. The idea to initiate these was based on the following justification:

Annual Plans: Five Year Plans, however carefully prepared and however firmly based, can be affected by unexpected events and by changes in the politico-economic situation. The main purpose of the Annual Plan would be to maintain the development effort during the year along the lines indicated in the Five Year Plan. The system of performance program budgeting, being introduced in the Central Government, should, through an appropriate linking of the physical and financial aspect of each program, help in strengthening the Annual Plan formulation process.

State Plans: In the States, Plan documents have been generally drawn upon the lines suggested by the Planning Commission. Necessarily there are many aspects of Plan formulation, which need attention after the process of the formal adoption of a State Plan has been concluded. Every State will have to undertake an analysis of fiscal and regulatory policies, administrative organizations and institutional framework at various levels.

District Planning: If the State Plans are to succeed, their formulation in relation to physical features and resources and the institutional organizations in each area is the first requirement. Development needs not only financial resources and material inputs but, personnel and the right kind of institutions. This requirement has to be worked out for each operational area. The natural corollary of beginning to plan realistically and from the bottom is to recognize that planning is not something that comes from outside or the above but what each State, district, locality and community does to develop its own resources and potentialities.

With regards to **Health Education**, the fourth plan stated that Education Bureau in States and at the Centre would effectively coordinate Health Education promotion activities. It is necessary that health care facilities are supported by an improved health information system. The machinery in States and at the Centre would be adequately streamlined to ensure a systematic review and evaluation of the on-going programs[23].

The **Fifth Five Year Plan** declared that country has adopted the policy 'Health for all by 2000 AD' enunciated in Alma Ata Declaration in 1977. The strategy to be followed over a period of 20 years up-to 2000 AD, based on the recommendation of the Working

Group on Health, will be as follows: Emphasis would be shifted from development of city based curative service's and super-specialties to tackling rural health problems. A rural health care system based on a combination of preventive, promotive and curative health care services would be built up starting from the village as the base[24].

The **Sixth Five Year Plan** mainly focused upon the decline of sex ratio and said that despite all these development measures and the Constitutional legal guarantees, women have lagged behind men in almost all sectors. There has been a steady decline in sex ratio. For 1,000 men there were 972 women in 1901, which became 946 in 1951 and 930 in 1971, while the position is opposite in the developed countries. The surveys by the Registrar-General of India revealed that the infant mortality rate (IMR) was more among female babies as compared to males in rural and urban areas[25]. It was during this plan the most significant step was taken, adoption of the National Health Policy by both Houses of Parliament. Health Care Programmes were restructured and reoriented towards this policy. Priority was given to extension and expansion of the rural health infrastructure through a network of community health centers, primary health centers and sub-centers, on a liberalized population norm. High priority was given to the development of primary health care located as close to the people as possible.

The **Seventh Five Year Plan** stated that one major problem in education and health is that of improving the quality. An improvement in the educational and health status of the poor will have a wide-ranging impact on the whole development process. Therefore, systematic attention to the quality and usefulness of the service provided at so large a cost to the public exchequer is necessary. With regards to the Health Education it was for the first time that the terminology of **Information, Education and Communication (IEC)** was used in the plan. It stated that the progress made so far in the promotion of Health Education is far from satisfactory. Efforts in the Seventh Plan were basically directed to develop and strengthen Health Education as an essential component of health services in the country. This was supported by adequate budgetary provision. It emphasized upon the efforts for the active use of different types of media to create awareness among the people and motivate them to utilize health services and to adopt healthful practices[26].

The plan declared that to achieve the national long-term demographic goals, educating and enlightening people on the benefits of late marriage and its social enforcement will have to be greatly emphasized. Special programs and incentives oriented towards eligible couples, particularly in the younger age-groups, were needed. Vigorous steps were to be taken to reduce maternal mortality as more than two-thirds of the women in the rural areas were still being attended to at childbirth by untrained Dais and there is, therefore, the Dais training program was augmented. Efforts were made to improve and upgrade the Management and Information, Education and Communication (IEC) skills of various categories of personnel, to identify the training needs, to strengthen the capabilities of various institutes at the state, regional and central levels and at the national level a consortium of premier management institutions with National Institute of Health and Family Welfare as a focal point to coordinate and undertake training activities was planned. Allocation of funds for IEC activities would be regulated in an appropriate manner and not be only confined to agencies like the Ministry of Information and Broadcasting, and Directorate of Audio-Visual Publicity. The strategies and channels would be diversified for better and more effective educational coverage.

The **Eighth Five Year Plan** for the first time focused upon "Human Development" and stated it as the ultimate goal of the Plan. It is towards this that employment generation, population control, literacy, education, health, drinking water and provision of adequate food and basic infrastructure were listed as the priorities. With regards to health it stated that the "Health for All" (HFA) paradigm must take into account not only the high risk vulnerable groups, i.e., mother and child (as done so far) but must also focus sharply on the underprivileged segments within the vulnerable groups. The National Health Policy (1983) reiterated India's commitment to attain "Health for All (HFA) by 2000 A.D".

The plan accepted that due to inadequacy of Information, Education and Communication (IEC) activities the knowledge of the community about the contraceptives, their availability, safety, etc. are at a low level, the IEC activities were directed more to national issues rather than personal issues. With this background, a future strategy was drawn, Information, Education and Communication, as critical inputs were to be strengthened and expanded. The IEC activities of the Health and the Family Welfare sector were integrated. The entire system of pricing the media time vis-à-vis its social responsibility were given a fresh look, different from the commercial angle area specific IEC material was to be developed and produced. The backbone of the IEC efforts, however, was grass-root level female worker to be trained and effectively utilized[27].

The **Ninth Five Year Plan** recognized the special health needs of women and the girl child and the importance of enhancing easy access to primary health care. There were many indicators to point out that the neglect of health needs of women especially that of the pregnant women, adolescent girls and girl-babies, was responsible for the present high rates of IMR/CMR/MMR. Therefore, a holistic approach with Reproductive Child Health (RCH) measures was adopted in improving the health status of women by focusing on their age-specific needs[28]. Improvement in the health status of women received high priority during the Eighth Plan. The erstwhile program of Maternal and Child Health services was recast as the Child Survival and Safe Motherhood (CSSM) program and launched in 72 districts during 1992-93. The same was further expanded to cover 466 districts by the end of the Eighth Plan.

Under CSSM training, 22715 medical officers and 92365 para medical workers were trained till September, 1996. These services of Child Survival and Safe Motherhood, as revealed by various evaluation studies, have contributed significantly to the reduction of Infant Mortality Rate from 79 to 72; Crude Birth Rate from 29.2 to 27.5 and Crude Death Rate from 10 to 9.0 during 1992 to 1996. An extensive network of 2424 Community Health Centres, 22,962 Primary Health Centres and 1,36,815 village level Sub-Centres was in actual operation by 1997 to extend primary health care services including safe motherhood and other family planning services to women in rural areas[29].

The **Tenth Five Year Plan** focuses upon the women of the country as an independent target group. It mentions: Girl children in the age group 0-14 years, deserve special attention because of the gender bias and discrimination they suffer from at the tender age. Adolescent girls in the age group 15-19 years are very sensitive from the viewpoint of planning because of the preparatory stage for their future productive and reproductive roles in the society and family respectively; and Women in the reproductive age 15-44 year need special care and attention because of their reproductive needs[30].

The Plan also quotes the National Health Policy 2001 (draft), which promises to ensure increased access to women to basic health care and commits highest priority to funding of the identified programs relating to women's health. During the Ninth Five Year Plan, the focus with regards to women's health shifted from the individualized vertical interventions to a more holistic integrated life-cycle approach with more attention to reproductive health care.

The **Tenth Five Year Plan** reflects the findings of the National Family Health Survey (NFHS) II of 1998-99, which showed that while 1.9 per cent of the adolescent married girls suffer from severe anemia, 45.9 per cent from moderate anemia. If left undetected and untreated, this will lead not only to increased morbidity amongst mothers, but also to higher risk of low birth rate and higher pre-natal mortality.

The Tenth Five Year Plan commits to improve the accessibility and utilization of services of primary health care and family welfare with a special focus on the under-served and the under-privileged segments of the population through universalizing of RCH services. Efforts have been planned to promote ready access to medical termination of pregnancy facilities and intra-partum care at PHCs, mainly to effectively enforce the Pre-natal Diagnostic Techniques (Regulation and prevention of use) Act, 1994.

IV. Certain Reflections

The evolution of Public Health Policies show a slow but steady learning from pilot projects and evaluation of implementation processes. A variety of methodological approaches have been adopted by policy analysts in doing so. These range from more formal approaches – such as macro economic growth models, cost benefit analysis, survey research, simulation models for generating demographic scenarios and action research to less structure field observations and consensus building through committees. Major changes in policy directions have emerged from a dialogue between different actors through a committee process. International professional opinion, especially through the WHO, played an important role in pushing innovative ideas within the government. Interestingly enough the facts that many of these new ideas were well demonstrated by private voluntary organizations in India provided further legitimacy to innovative policy and program initiatives[31].

To date the impact of Family Planning programs have been measured mainly in terms of its contribution to increase contraceptive prevalence and to decrease fertility. These indicators are inadequate for measuring impact of Reproductive Health program and therefore new indicators for monitoring Reproductive Health services and service quality from the perspective of the client were urgently needed. Providing comprehensive RH service to all is a desirable goal, however since there is a considerable variability in the organizational capacity of programs in the different regions and states of India, the extent to which a program might extend without compromising the quality of effectiveness of existing service must be seriously considered, there is a clear need to prioritize and develop a phased approach with an incremental addition of health interventions that require greater skills and resources[32]. The proponents of the Reproductive Health framework believe that Reproductive Health is inextricably linked to the subject of reproductive rights and freedom and to women's status and empowerment. Thus the Reproductive Health approach extends beyond the narrow confines of the Family Planning. To encompass all aspects of human sexuality and Reproductive Health needs during the various stages of the life cycle in addressing the needs of both women and men, such an approach places an emphasis on developing programs that enable clients to make informed choices, receive screening counseling services and education for responsible and healthy sexuality, access services for preventing unwanted pregnancy, safe abortion, maternity care and child survival and for the prevention and management of reproductive morbidity. Thus RH programs are concerned with a set of specific health problems, identifiable clusters of client groups and distinctive goals and strategies[33]

Some of the serious Reproductive Health issues in India demand extreme concern. Here, abortion can be legally sought on broad health grounds, in case deformities are detected in the foetus, when the pregnancy is the consequence of rape, and also in the event of contraceptive failure. Despite the legal status of abortion in India, an estimated 4.5 million illegal abortions were carried out annually as of 1992. For every legally induced abortion, there were 10-11 that were performed in unlicensed facilities or by unqualified health workers. Between 11-14% of all maternal deaths in rural India during 1990-94 were reported to be caused by abortion complications. Sixty per cent of all abortion deaths in 1994 were in young women 15-24 years of age. India has been the only country where anemia emerges as an important factor in maternal deaths, where almost a fifth of all deaths (19.3%) were reported to be related to anaemia. One of the earliest and most often quoted community-based studies on gynecological morbidity was done in rural Maharashtra by Bang et al (1989). This study, which combined self –reporting with clinical and laboratory examination, found 55% of 650 women included in the study to have gynecological complaints, while 45% were symptom free. Of those who had gynecological complaints, 92% had one or more clinically verifiable "gynecological or sexual diseases", with an average of 3.6 diseases per woman. Results from similar studies in rural West Bengal, Mumbai, Baroda, rural Karnataka and rural Gujarat, show the prevalence of gynecological morbidity to vary from 26% to 74%[34].

It needs to be asserted here that, biologically, women are more susceptible to most STIs than men. This is because of the shape of the vagina and a greater mucosal surface exposed to a greater quantity of pathogens during sexual intercourse, since the quantity of seminal fluid is far greater than the vaginal fluid involved. High prevalence rates of and at the same time lack of information on RTIs and STDs affirms the opinion that reproductive morbidity and mortality amongst Indian women is mainly a result of lack of health education along with many other causes like poverty, powerlessness, low social status, malnutrition, infection, high fertility and lack of access to health care. Application of IEC strategies with a continuous follow up and counseling can be the only best way to reduce the same.

Health Education, therefore, is essential to help individuals, groups, communities and especially to women "to become competent in, and to carry on those activities they must undertake for themselves, in order to realize fully a complete state of health". The preamble of the Constitution of the World Health Organization recognized this and included two relevant principles. One was: "The extension to all peoples of the benefits of medical, psychological and related knowledge is essential to the fullest attainment of health". Another was: "Informed opinion and active cooperation on the part of the public are of utmost importance in the improvement of the health of the people." This early concern of the Organization has been reiterated in the resolutions of the World Health Assembly, the Executive Board, and the Regional Committee for South-East Asia, and reflected in the Fifth and Sixth General Programs of Work. In 1974, the twenty-seventh World Health Assembly recommended that Health Education activities should be intensified in all WHO programs. It also requested the Organization to enlarge its support to interested Member States in strengthening the planning, implementation and evaluation of the Health Education components of their National Health programs[35].

With such decisions however, films, cinema slides, exhibits, radio, newspapers and other mass media, were utilized, which provided health information to the public. Such activities were sporadic, and not closely related to the educational efforts of health workers in the different health services. The result was, the public largely remained passive spectators of these programs.

Policy and program issues are entwined and it is not enough to deal with only one set of issues. Some observers have expressed concern that focusing on programmatic issues in Reproductive Health and Family Planning will fail because doing so deals narrowly with a subset of issue about the health delivery system and does not confront the fundamental social issues that engender high fertility as well as persistent poverty[36].

The RCH program initiated since the year 1996 envisages changes not only at policy level but also in management and implementation of the program. Besides the removal of targets, other policy changes relate to encouraging the states to remove in a phased manner, the incentive payments to both providers and acceptors of certain family planning methods; shifting financial priorities from further build-up of infrastructure to increased sustainability and use of existing facilities; expanding access by encouraging the use of NGOs and the private sector to fill gaps in the public sector services.

Program level changes include: district-level planning and monitoring that is more responsive to local needs; improved quality of care and increased client focus; expanded community involvement and responsibility for the Health and Family welfare through the decentralized system of government (Panchayati Raj); and the improved referral system for the health care seekers. At the service delivery level, the changes include revitalization of the existing network of rural health facilities through better supplies of drugs and equipment, training and better information and counseling for clients and communities.

Some efforts such as Information, education and Communication (IEC), training and program monitoring were nation-wide, whereas some interventions were incorporated only in selected districts. Even within the districts, the interventions were to be introduced in a progressively phased manner on the basis of the existing institutional capacity and Reproductive Health needs of the population in the blocks or sub-district units. Besides addressing the issues of quality and informed choice, the RCH project provides a vehicle for continued policy dialogue; continued evaluation and reviews; and significant flexibility for implementing recommendations of the evaluations and reviews through annual and state-specific modifications to implementation plans. While the details of the RCH project document can be debated and discussed, it does address several issues that have been neglected in India's Family Welfare Program[37].

With the present socio economic framework of the country, and the health status of women resulting from early marriage and early childbearing, IEC efforts aiming at increase in the age of marriage and childbearing, spacing of births through contraception, permanent methods like Vasectomy emphasizing upon male involvement, prevention and cure for RTIs and STIs, and emphasis on sanitation and hygiene are needed to ensure sound Reproductive Health. Women need to be educated regarding a long range of complications like anemia, infection, pre-eclampsia, malpresentation and obstructed labour and should be made aware about the danger signs of pregnancy, knowledge regarding breast feeding, nutrition, and immunization. Further to this it is equally important to educate women on the services available and the areas to seek help and information and special efforts are needed to promote male responsibility and enhance the involvement of men.

For undertaking the abovementioned efforts outreach services should be strengthened to ensure that all women are registered as early in pregnancy as possible and antenatal care initiated, in addition PHC's must also be upgraded to manage some complication and provide facilities and delivery[38].

A change in focus from a top down population control driven approach to a gender sensitive, client based approach to address Reproductive Health needs through the implementation of RCH program based on CNA approach has been initiated in 1996-97. A number of schemes and programs have been designed at national and state levels to enhance access and improve the quality of services with a special focus on women. However, one needs to look at the demographic and health profile of the country, which is not uniform. The examination of the state wide data regarding behaviour of the important demographic and health indicators shows very clearly that any operational strategy to be successful will have to be based on disaggregated and region specific approach. The classic example can be quoted of four states of Bihar, MP, Rajasthan and UP which constitute about 40% of the country's population have IMR and MMR levels distinctly higher than the national average. Special area development projects have been already been launched in these states with the help of World Bank, UNFPA and other funding agencies[39].

It is also necessary to note that policies are implemented without recognizing the organizational and resource requirements for implementing them. While comprehensive Population or Health Policies are evolved, the necessary organizational forms and processes are not created. Thus, an adequate appreciation of the implementation aspect and the neglect of structural and resource constraints contribute to the ultimate ineffectiveness of policies. The capability of health programs to effectively reach the vast majority of the rural masses depends on the quality, distribution of health manpower. It has been felt that while India is rich in both policy and analytical expertise, it is rather poor in policy analysis. Reasons for this situation have been attributed to the demand and supply aspects of the equation. The government, it has been argued is not sufficiently interested in promoting or encouraging policy analysis. It does not part with the data, act upon the results of analysis or encourage the wider dissemination of research findings. The complaints from the other side are that the academic community is ignorant or disinterested in the working of the government, is shy of attacking practical problems and tends to take refuge[40].

When method-specific targets were removed abruptly nationwide, the change shook the system. Several critics questioned the rationale behind the action, pointing to a decline in program performance in the first year as evidence that the move was ill-advised. However, studies have quoted that contraceptive prevalence has not declined and clients report greater satisfaction with services. "The mantra of quality has been sanctified at the field level," but there is room for further improvement. Services for emergency obstetric care, safe abortion, and treatment of reproductive tract infections and infertility are still not in place. Health services for adolescent girls have a special significance in India, where there is a strong son preference and where adolescent pregnancy is the norm. About 85 per cent of adolescent girls and adult women in India are anemic; the association between anemia and low birth weight, premature birth, and perinatal and maternal death is confirmed and a dearth of information on how to manage the needs of adolescents, and that young people must be brought in as equal partners in designing policies and programs to address their needs. For the most part, reproductive health initiatives have targeted women. However, because men make the majority of sexual and reproductive health decisions in India, "men's involvement as responsible partners is essential." Furthermore, men have reproductive and sexual health needs of their own that should be addressed.

Reproductive health is related to sexual health in particular and to sexuality in general. Past programs skirted these issues because of political and cultural sensitivity. The reluctance to discuss these issues has limited the effectiveness of programs designed to improve women's health, promote family planning, and prevent the transmission of HIV and other sexually transmitted infections. Because past programs focused mainly on birth control, many reproductive health problems were ignored. Recent efforts to implement the essential package of reproductive health services have underscored the complexity of diagnosing and treating reproductive tract infections in women.

The momentum achieved by the new program has been significant, but many challenges lie ahead. In a country as diverse as India, there will never be a single blueprint for family planning and reproductive health policy. The first important task, to change policy in the largest democracy in the world — has been accomplished. India is now on the threshold of change as it puts the new agenda into effect. Partnerships must be forged between the government and the civil society to create the synergy needed for promoting social change, for it is that which will eventually determine the success of these endeavors[41].

Apart from this, implementing the Reproductive Health approach requires increasing the community's involvement in an ownership of population issues at all levels of program design and implementation. India's present policy approach emphasizes the opportunity provided by the Panchayati Raj to decentralize the program design and management by placing responsibility with the Panchayats, the Nagarpalikas, and the Zilla Parishads, thereby developing locally relevant approaches for program implementation[42].

REFERENCES

1. Government of India, *Report of Independent Commission on Health in India*, New Delhi, 1984, p. 320.

2. Phyllis Tilson Piotrow, D. Lawrence Kincaid, Jose G. Rimon II, & Ward Rinehart, *Health Communication – Lessons form Family Planning and Reproductive Health*, (Johns Hopkins School of Public Health, Praeger Publishers, 1997), p. 15.

3. *Ibid.*, p. 6.

4. Government of India, *National Health Policy 1983*, (New Delhi, India, Department of Family Welfare, Govt. of India, 1983).

5. Government of India, *National Population Policy 2000*, (New Delhi, India, Department of Family Welfare, Govt. of India, 2000).

6. Communication Strategies As Stated in the *Programme of Action adopted* At the ICPD, Cairo, 5-13 September 1994.
7. Government of India, *Towards Equality* - Report of the Committee on the Status of Women in India, New Delhi, 1974, p. 325.
8. Peter Mayer, 'Data and Perspectives, India's Falling Sex ratios', *Population and Development Review*, Vol. 25, No. 2, June 99, p. 323.
9. Anthony Measham and Richard Heaver, *Supplement to India's Family Welfare Program-Moving to Reproductive and Child Health Approach*, Washington the World Bank, 1996 p. 33.
10. *Towards Equality*, n. 7, p. 314.
11. *Towards Equality*, n. 7, p. 325.
12. *Annual Report*, (Office of Registrar General, India and Ministry of Health and Family Welfare, New Delhi, 2002), Chapter 1 – Perspective.
13. *Annual Report*, (Office of Registrar General, India and Ministry of Health and Family Welfare, New Delhi, 2002), Chapter – 07: Information Education and Communication.
14. Karen Hardee, Kokila Agarwal, Nancy Luke, Ellen Wilson, Margaret Pendzich, Marguerite Farrell, Harry Cross, *Post Cairo Reproductive Health Policies and Programs: A Comparative Study of Eight Countries*, (Washington DC, USAID, 1998).
15. Phyllis Tilson Piotrow and Jose G. Rimon II, 'Population Program', *Asia Pacific Population Journal*, Vol. 14, No. 4,1999, p. 73-90.
16. *Ibid.*
17. Quoted in Phyllis Tilson Piotrow, D. Lawrence Kincaid, Jose G. Rimon II, & Ward Rinehart, "Health Communication – Lessons for Family Planning and Reproductive Health", Johns Hopkins School of Public Health, USA, Praeger Publishers, 1997. p. 8.
18. Government of India, *Tenth Five Year Plan*, (New Delhi, Planning Commission, 2002), Col. 2.11.2.
19. Government of India, *First Five Year Plan*, (New Delhi, Planning Commission,,1951), Chapter 32.
20. *Ibid.*
21. Government of India, *Second Five Year Plan*, (New Delhi, Planning Commission 1956).
22. Government of India, *Third Five Year Plan*, (New Delhi, Planning Commission 1961).
23. Government of India, *Fourth Five Year Plan*, (New Delhi, Planning Commission 1966).

24. Government of India, *Fifth Five Year Plan*, (New Delhi, Planning Commission, 1974).

25. Government of India, *Sixth Five Year Plan*, (New Delhi, Planning Commission 1980).

26. Government of India, *Seventh Five Year Plan*, (New Delhi, Planning Commission 1985).

27. Government of India, *Eighth Five Year Plan*, (New Delhi, Planning Commission 1992).

28. Government of India, *Ninth Five Year Plan*, (New Delhi, Planning Commission 1997), Vol. II – 3.8.30

29. Government of India, Ninth Five Year Plan – Vol. II – 3.8.61, New Delhi, Planning Commission 1997.

30. Government of India, *Tenth Five Year Plan*, (New Delhi, Planning Commission 2002).

31. R.S. Ganpathy, S.R. Ganesh, Rushikesh Maru, Samuel Paul, Ram Mohan Rao, *Public Policy and Policy Analysis in India*, (New Delhi, Sage Publications, 1985), p. 10.

32 Saroj Pachauri, *Defining a Reproductive Health Package for India: A.Proposed Framework, South and East Asia*, Regional Working Papers, (New Delhi, The Population Council,1995), p. 8.

34. World Health Organization, Regional Office, South East Asia, *Women of South East Asia – A Health Profile*, (New Delhi, 2000) , pp. 75-97, 200–208.

35. World Health Organization, *A Decade of Health Development in South-East Asia-1968-77*, (Regional Office, South East Asia, New Delhi, 1978), pp. 34, 112, 139-147.

36. Anthony Measham and Richard Heaver n. 9, p. 19.

37. Health Watch Trust, *The Community Needs Based RCH in India: Progress and Constraints*, Jaipur, 1999. p. 3-5.

38. Saroj Pachauri, n. 32, p. 32.

39. Anthony Measham and Richard Heaver, n. 9, p. 3.

40. R.S. Ganpathy, S.R. Ganesh, Rushikesh Maru, Samuel Paul, Ram Mohan Rao , n. 31, p. 250.

41 Saroj Pachauri *Implementing a Reproductive Health Agenda in India: The Beginning*, (New Delhi).

42 Anthony Measham and Richard Heaver, n.9, pp. 22-23.

5

Administrative Structures; Information Education and Communication Programs in Melghat Region

Introduction

The present chapter focuses upon: Administrative structures of the Central and Maharashtra State Government for implementation of Public Health programs and information about the programs; Information, Education and Communication (IEC) efforts and programs undertaken by the State IEC Bureau; and Public Health schemes implemented by the Maharashtra State Government, with special reference to the Melghat region of Amravati district.

Administrative Structures of the Central and Maharashtra State Government for Implementation of Public Health Programs

Central Government

As mentioned earlier, Health being a "State Subject", the responsibility for the implementation of all health programs rests with the respective State governments. The Center is, however, responsible in both the legislative and executive fields for international health, standards of medical education, and for developing central agencies and institutions for the promotion of research and training.

The Central and State Governments, have responsibilities for the prevention of infectious diseases, mental deficiency, poisons and dangerous drugs, collection of vital statistics and prevention of food adulteration. At the Central level, the Ministry of Health and Family Welfare is responsible to the Government for all health matters. Executive authority is vested in the Secretary of Health and Family Welfare. The Ministry is responsible for maintaining liaison with allied ministries, international organizations and other autonomous bodies. If formulates the National Policy on Health and Family Welfare. There is a **Central Council of Health and Family Welfare,** which includes representatives of State Health Ministries and other high level officers from the Center and States. It is presided over by the Minister of Health and Family Welfare and usually meets annually to take policy decisions. The administrative structure of State Health Services is similar to that of the Central Health Ministry. In each district, there is a District Health Organization headed by a District Health Officer or a Civil Surgeon, assisted by other officers.

The basic health unit within the district is the Primary Health Center (PHC), one per Community Development Block, each having a number of sub-centers. Each PHC covers the health needs of a varying number of villages (150-350) and a population of approximately 30,000. The main functions of the PHC are: medical care; control of communicable diseases; environmental sanitation; Maternal and Child Health services including Family Welfare, school health, immunization, Health Education, and registration of vital statistics. In March 1977 there were 5380 primary health centers and 38110 sub-centers providing basic health services to the rural population. Apart from this, a number of National Programs for the eradication of communicable diseases are in operation.

In 1952 India was the first country in the world to launch a National Program emphasizing Family Planning to the extent necessary for reducing birth rates "to stabilize the population at a level consistent with the requirement of national economy". After 1952, sharp decline in death rates were, however not accompanied by a similar drop in birth rates. The National Health Policy, 1983 stated that replacement level of total fertility rate (TFR) should be achieved by the year 2000.

Table 5.1

India's demographic achievement Half a century after formulation of the National Family Welfare Program, India has:

- Reduced crude birth rate (CBR) from 40.8 (1951) to 26.4 (1998, SRS);
- Halved the infant mortality rate (IMR) from 146 per 1000 live birth(1951) to 72 per 1000 live birth (1998,SRS);
- Quadrupled the couple protection rate (CPR) from 10.4% (1971) to 44% (1999);
- Reduced crude death rate (CDR) from 25(1951) to 9.0 (1998, SRS);
- Added 25 years to life expectancy from 37 years to 62 years;
- Achieved nearly universal awareness of need for and methods of family planning; and
- Reduced total fertility rate from 6.0 (1951) to 3.3(1997, SRS)

Source: ***National Population Policy 2000*** **(Government of India).**

The National Population Policy – 2000 [1] provides a policy framework for advancing goals and prioritizing strategies during the next decade to meet the Reproductive and Child Health needs of the people of India, and to achieve net replacement level (TFR) by 2010. It is based upon the need to simultaneously address issues of child survival, maternal health, and contraception, while increasing out reach and coverage of a comprehensive package of RCH services by government, industry and the voluntary non-governmental sector, working in partnership.

Programs for safe motherhood, Universal Immunization, Child Survival and Oral Re-hydration, have been combined into an integrated Reproductive and Child Health Program, which also includes promoting management of STIs and RTIs. Information, Education and Communication (IEC) of Family Welfare messages will be disseminated to the remote corners of the country, in local dialects, ensuring that the messages are effectively conveyed. These need to be strengthened and their outreach widened, with locally relevant, and locally comprehensible media and messages on the model of the total literacy campaigns, which have successfully mobilized local population related issues, via artists, popular film stars, doctors, vaidyas, hakims, nurses, local midwives, women's organization, and youth organizations.

A **National Commission on Population** presided over by the Prime Minister, has the Chief Ministers of all States and Union Territories, and the Central Minister in-charge of the Department of Family Welfare and other concerned Central Ministries and Departments. To enhance performance, particularly in states with currently below average socio-demographic indices that need focused attention, a **Technology Mission in the Department of Family Welfare** was to be established to provide technology support in respect of design and monitoring of projects and programs for RCH, as well as for IEC campaigns.

The promotional and motivational measures to be undertaken:

1. Panchayat and Zila Parishads to be rewarded and honoured for exemplary performance in universalizing the small family norm, achieving reductions in infant mortality and birth rates, and promoting literacy with completion of primary schooling.
2. The Balika Samriddhi Yojana run by the Department of Women and Child Development to promote survival and care of the girl child, will continue. A cash incentive of Rs. 500 is awarded at the birth of the girl child of birth order 1 or 2.
3. Maternity Benefit Scheme run by the Department of Rural Development to continue. A cash incentive of Rs. 500 is awarded to mothers who have their first child after 19 years of age, for birth of the first or second child only. Disbursement of the cash award will in future be linked to compliance with ante-natal check up, institutional delivery by trained birth attendant, registration of birth, and BCG immunization.
4. A Family Welfare linked Health Insurance Plan to be established. Couples below the poverty line, who undergo sterilization with not more than two living children, would become eligible (along with children) for health insurance (for hospitalization) not exceeding Rs. 5000, and a personal accident insurance cover for the spouse undergoing sterilization.
5. Couples below the poverty line who marry after the legal age of marriage, register the marriage, have their first child after the mother reaches the age of 21, accept the small family norm, and adopt a terminal method after the birth of the second child, will be rewarded.

6. A revolving fund to be set up for income-generating activities by village-level Self Help Groups, who provide community-level health care services.
7. Crèches and child care centers to be opened in rural areas and urban slums. This will facilitate and promote participation of women in paid employment.
8. A wider, affordable choice of contraceptives to be made accessible at diverse delivery points, with counseling services to enable acceptors to exercise voluntary and informed consent.
9. Facilities for safe abortion to be strengthened and expanded.
10. Products and services to be made affordable through innovative social marketing schemes.
11. Local entrepreneurs at village levels to be provided soft loans and encouraged to run ambulance services to supplement the existing arrangements for referral transportation.
12. Increased vocational training schemes for girls, leading to self-employment to be encouraged.
13. Strict enforcement of Child Marriage Restraint Act, 1976.
14. Strict enforcement of the Pre-Natal Diagnostic Techniques Act 1996.
15. Soft loans to ensure mobility of the ANMs to be increased.

Support community activities such as dissemination of IEC material including leaflets and posters, and promotion of folk jatras, songs and dances to promote healthy mother and healthy baby messages, along with good management practices to ensure safe motherhood including early recognition of danger signs were proposed.

The RCH Programme is a composite program incorporating, inter alia, the inputs of the Government of India as well as funding support from external donor agencies including World Bank and the European Commission. It has been taken up in recognition of the legitimate right of the citizens to be provided with all the facilities for Reproductive and Child Health. The RCH Program incorporates the components of the Child Survival and Safe Motherhood Programme and further includes two additional components- one relating to sexually transmitted diseases (STD) and the other relating to reproductive tract infection (RTI).

The importance of IEC activity cannot be overstated for demystifying the RCH and population issues among public and in advocacy role. Imaginatively produced programs have a very strong persuasive effect. Therefore, the department of Family Welfare has been implementing a large IEC programme under which extensive use is being made of Doordarshan, All India Radio, Directorate of Advertising and Visual Publicity, Directorate of Field publicity, Song and Drama division and Films Division under the Ministry of Information and Broadcasting. In addition, Mahila Swasthya Sanghs, sensitization of opinion leaders, health awareness units in Nehru Yuvak Kendras are being supported.

Maharashtra: Pattern of Panchayati Raj[2]

Based on the recommendations of the Naik Committee, Maharashtra adopted the Panchayati Raj pattern, which deviated from the model laid down by the Balwantrai Mehta Study Team by making the district body – the Zilla Parishad a strong executive body at the district level rather than the block level body. Accordingly, the Maharashtra Zilla Parishads and Panchayats Act were enacted, which created two tiers – Zilla Parishad and Panchayat Samiti – since the Village Panchayats were already working under the Bombay Village Panchayats Act, 1958. Though the Naik Committee recommended a three-tier structure, consisting of the Zilla Parishad, Panchayat Samiti and Village panchayat, it gave Zilla Parishads and not the Panchayat Samiti the central place; recommended direct, instead of indirect, elections at the district level (Since then this has been amended and any voter can contest for membership to the Panchayat Samiti); did not give legislators ex-officio status on the district level body; and kept the District Collector outside the Panchayati Raj System. It also sought to place the district officials responsible for development under the control of the Zilla Parishad.

A Dual control operates wherein the District Health Officer like other development officers is directly under the control of the Chief Executive Officer and also his Health cadre officers in the Health Directorate of the State Government. The Act has also given powers to the State Government to provide support and direction and exercise suitable supervision and control in regard to the working of the Panchyati Raj. One of the principal features of the

Panchayati Raj in Maharashtra has been the separation of the executive function from the deliberative function. The policy making function has been entrusted to the elected representatives of the people. One third of the elected seats at all the three levels of the Panchayati Raj are reserved for women who can give a push to the Health of women and children. Similarly, elected seats are reserved for the S.C. and S.T. as per legal provisions.

To provide democratic direction and the necessary supervision and support to the planning and execution of various types of civic services and development schemes and works approved by the Zilla Parishad, a Standing Committee and nine Subject Committees – one of which is the Health Committee, as provided statutorily, have been set up by the Zilla Parishad. The secretary to the Health Committee is the District Health Officer. The Committee meets every month and policy decisions related to health development in the district are taken.

Each Community Development Block has a Panchayat Samiti. The Chairman of the Samiti is vested with both financial and administrative powers under the Act. The administrative powers comprise conducting and regulating meetings of the Samiti, exercising supervision and control over the work of the Block Development Officer and other officers and employees of the Panchayat Samiti. His/Her financial powers relate to the sanctioning of certain development schemes financed from the Block Grants and also accepting tenders or contracts related to development schemes of costs lying within the legally prescribed limits. The Deputy Chairman presides over the meetings of the Samiti in the absence of the Chairman and also performs duties delegated to him/her by the chairman under prescribed rules. He is also responsible for the inspection of working progress or any institution financed or under the jurisdiction of the Zilla Parishad and situated within the Samiti area and send his/her report to the Chairman who has similar powers.

The Block Development Officer (BDO) is the Chief Executive Officer of the Samiti and is appointed by the State Government. Normally, she/he is drawn from the State Government's newly created Maharashtra Development Service, which is analogous to the State's Civil Service. He acts as an ex-officio Secretary of the Samiti and attends its meetings, provides any information needed by members and maintains Samiti's records. She/He is generally responsible to the Chairman of the Samiti for her/his official decisions and actions, though administratively she/he is under the control of the Chief Executive Officer of the Zilla Parishad. As an executive head of the Samiti administration, she/he is responsible for ensuring the implementation of the Samiti approved development works and schemes as well as the maintenance of the completed ones. She/He is also responsible for the implementation of schemes and works entrusted by the Zilla Parishad or the State Government to the Samiti.

The Gram Panchayat is composed of 7 to 15 members, depending upon the size of its coverage of population. The members are directly elected on the basis of adult franchise. One-third of the seats are reserved for women and there is reservation of seats for SC/ST in proportion to their population. The Sarpanch (Chairman) is elected by the members and is responsible for ensuring that the Panchayat is functioning in accordance with the provision in the Bombay Village Panchayat Act 1958, decisions of the Panchayat, directives of the Zilla Parishad, Panchayat Samiti and the State Government. Any views expressed in the Gram Sabha (Village Assembly) have to be considered by the Panchayat and the Sarpanch. A Secretary-cum-village Level Worker (VLW) appointed by the Zilla Parishad and carrying out both administrative and developmental function assists him.

Background of Public Health

The Public Health Department of Maharashtra state has a history of almost 150 years. It is interesting to look into the process of its development. It started functioning as a "Vaccination Department" way back in 1858, later, in the year 1895, with addition of a few more functions it was re-designated as "Sanitary Department" with Sanitary Commissioner as its Chief. This department was general, with its headquarters at Bombay. The year 1921 heralded the establishment of "Directorate of Public Health". It had three posts of Assistant Director, one each for the three, North, South and East divisions in the erstwhile Bombay in the year 1941.

It was around this time, the concept of comprehensive health care was advocated by Bhore Committee. The shift in emphasis from curative to preventive services necessitated many changes in the pattern o delivery of Health Services. The Urban oriented approach was transformed into a rural oriented one. The Bhore Committtee recommended creation of a network of Primary Health Centers to bring health services nearer to the rural people. The launching of Community Development program in the year 1952 must be regarded as an important landmark in the development of Health Services. Subsequently, Primary Health Centers were established in each block. Zilla Parishads were formed in 1962 and the overall responsibility of delivery of health care was transferred to the Zilla Parishads. The Directorate of Public Health and the office of the Surgeon General were first integrated and then reorganized into two separate Directorates in the year 1970, the Directorate of Health Services and the Directorate of Medical Education and Research. The headquarters of the Directorate of Public Health was also shifted to Mumbai. For supervision at divisional level, the Deputy Directors of Health Services in-charge Circles were located at seven circle headquarters, Mumbai, Pune, Aurangabad, Nagpur, Akola, Nasik and Kolhapur.

The year 1978 — the year of Alma Ata declaration and the National Health Policy formulated in 1983, triggered the "period of rapid expansion" of Health Services. The Health Services in Maharashtra responded fittingly to this commitment and the infrastructure presently available is a testimony of these efforts. The state has always remained in the forefront in implementing all the National Health Programs. New programs have been added from time to time to achieve our goal "Health For All.[3]

The Public Health Department in Maharashtra comprises of the Directorate of Health Services, Medical Education and Research, Directorate of ESIS, Directorate of Ayurveda, and Food and Drug Administration. The Directorate of Health Services prominently looks after Medical Help, Control of Communicable Diseases, Family Welfare, Maternal and Child Health, Preventive Hygiene, Services for Nutritional Supplementation, and Training of Medical Candidates. As per the requirement of the State, the Public Health department allocates finances for the following: Prevention and Control of Diseases, Urban Health Services through Hospitals, and Clinics, Family Welfare-Maternal and Child Health-School Education, Advice on Food and Nutrition and Health Education[4].

Rural Health, which is one of the important parts of Public Health department, comprises of various preventive programs. The financial allocation of these programs is as follows: Direction and Administration; Training; Prevention and Control of diseases; Production of serums and vaccines; Public Health Laboratory; Health Education and Publicity; Health transport; Malpraman- and hygiene; Grants-in-aid to Zilla Parishads; Health Statistics and Research.

Prevention and Control of the following epidemic diseases is an important program of health services: National program for control of blindness; Filaria control program; Plague control program; Malaria control program; Epidemic control program; Guinea worm eradication program; Leprosy control program; T.B. Control program; Goitre control program.

Table 5.2

Health Infrastructure in the State Referral Network

Sr. No.	*Particulars*	
1.	District Hospital	Secondary Referral
2.	First Referral Unit	First Referral
3.	Primary Health Centre	Per 30,000 Population
4.	Sub-Centre	Per 5,000 Population

Source: *Health Status, 2002* **(Public Health Department, Government of Maharashtra).**

Table 5.3

Health Personnel in the State:

Sr. No.	Particulars	
1.	MMHS Class I	1177
2.	MMHS Class II	5075
3.	GSS Class I	57
4.	GSS Class II	384
5.	Health Assistant (M)	4642
6.	Health Assistant (F)	3586
7.	MPW (M)	12646
8.	MPW (F)	11915
9.	Trained TBAs	45681

Source: ***Health Status*, 2002 (Public Health Department, Government of Maharashtra).**

See the following charts for details

Chart No. 1. Organizational structure of Public Health Department.

Chart No. 2. Organizational structure of Family Welfare Bureau.

State Government Programs in Public Health

1. *Hospital based services:* Today, the Public Health Department of Government of Maharashtra, provides for various services in the state and has established 16703 beds in different set ups through the program providing health facilities, out of which 6691 beds are available in district hospitals, 982 in maternity hospitals, 5795 in mental health centers, 795 in other government hospitals, 898 in cottage hospitals and 1622 in TB hospitals. Accordingly the department implements the following programs through the services in the hospitals: National Tuberculosis Control Program, Family Welfare Program, Intensive care for the new born and mental health centers.

2. *Super Specialty Services:* This comprises of Cardiac surgery, Nephrology, C.T. Scan, Paediatric surgery, Plastic surgery, Oncology and Trauma care.

3. *Cancer Prevention Program:* Under this program all the district hospitals and women's hospitals undertake the Pap Smear test for the diagnosis of the cervical cancer in women. Accordingly, all the lab technicians and the Medical Officers of the concerned hospitals have been trained for the same.
4. *Jeevandayi Arogya Yojana:* Under this scheme, the families Below Poverty Line (BPL) are provided with medical services for different types of diseases.
5. ***Manavi Avayava Pratiropan Kayada** (Human Organs Transplantation Act) –1994:* The present act has been made applicable since February 4, 1995.
6. *National AIDS Control Program:* The National AIDS Control Program has been converted into "Maharashtra State AIDS Control Society" since July 16, 1998 and is being run independently.
7. *Maharashtra Health Services Development Project:* In order to improve and upgrade the quality, capacity and utility of the state health services the state government has initiated the said project since January 9, 1999.
8. *National Mental Health Program:* The present program is meant for improving the services in the field of mental health and accordingly undertakes: training of officials from PHCs and Rural Hospitals; to provide with OPD for mental health in District Hospitals and Rural Hospitals; strengthening of Regional Mental Health Centers.
9. *Women Empowerment Program:* Some of the programs mainly meant for women like the Nav Sanjeevan scheme and Matrutva Anudan Yojana are undertaken under this program.

Maharashtra: State Policy for Reproductive Health

The Family Welfare Program in Maharashtra was initiated in 1957. As per the guidelines set by the Central Government, the program has been ongoing since then. With the aim of Health for All, the program of Child Survival and Safe Motherhood and Reproductive and Child Health program have been undertaken. Accordingly efforts are being undertaken for the reduction of birth rate, infant mortality rate, maternal mortality rate and death rate.

The established infrastructure and mechanisms of the urban and rural areas of the Public Health Department provide the following services: vasectomy, tubectomy, Intra Uterine Devices, oral contraception and condoms. The program is implemented through the Zilla Parishads of 33 districts and 15 Municipal Corporations. The program with an earlier target based approach has been changed to a target free approach in the year 1996-97, by the central government.

The implementation of the abovementioned program with the help of IEC techniques, information material, and personal meetings and counselling, the state has succeeded in achieving 52% of involvement of women in following various Family Planning methods. Apart from this the state has brought down the birth rate to 21.1 per thousand. Further the couple protection rate has increased, as well as spacing between two children has increased. The age of marriage has also increased.

In the year 1994, the ICPD at Cairo analyzed the reason for not reaching the goals set for Population Control. Subsequent sample studies indicated that there are some areas where the earlier program has not reached. Therefore, the entire strategy was changed and the following issues were given priority. Based on these priorities, the RCH program was formulated by Government of India. The State has accepted the strategy of implementing Reproductive and Child Health (RCH) program, which places a challenge to the health infrastructure since the components include comprehensive health care for all age groups. The issues like adolescent health, age at marriage, prenatal sex determination, sex education, unwanted pregnancy, women's empowerment, RTI/STI & HIV/AIDS need to be seriously addressed. The RCH program is implemented in the state since 1997. The program is monitored by the state Family Welfare Bureau, which is located at Pune.

Female ratio in Maharashtra State has come down to 922 compared to 934 in the 1991 census. The Supreme Court has already directed all the States to take stringent measures against the mal-utilization of the PNDT act. The Government of India has identified National Institute of Health & Family Welfare (NIHFW) as the Nodal Agency for Training activities under the RCH Program.

The State has formed the "State Level RCH Training Co-ordination Committee". According to the guidelines of NIHFW and in consultation with the Collaborating Training Institute (CTI) i.e. KEM Hospital & Research Centre, Pune, the Comprehensive Training Action Plan (CTP) has been prepared.

For implementing this program the following institutional arrangements have been made[5]:

Table 5.4

1.	Secretary level division	–	1
2.	Family welfare division of Directorate of Health Services, Mumbai	–	1
3.	State Family Welfare Bureau, Pune	–	1
4.	District family Welfare Bureau andSmall Family Welfare Bureau	–	29
5.	City Family Welfare Bureau, Mumbai, Pune, Solapur, Nagpur	–	7
6.	Rural Family Welfare Centers	–	433
7.	Urban Family Welfare Centers	–	74
8.	Rural Family Welfare Sub-Centers	–	1997
9.	Post-Partum care centers attached to rural hospitals	–	129
10.	Health Posts	–	280

Out of these following are being managed by Municipalities and NGOs

1. Rural Family Welfare Centers 5
2. Urban Family Welfare Centers 54
3. Post Partum care centers attached to the hospitals 40

Activities under Maternal and Child Health Program

Immunization of mothers and children.

Scheme of Prophylaxis against blindness due to Vitamin 'A' deficiency in children.

Scheme of Prophylaxis Nutritional Anemia in Mothers and Children.

Scheme of Typhoid and Polio Immunization of Children in Maharashtra state.

The major head program wise details of total budget estimates are:

Direction and administration

Training

Rural Family Welfare Services

Urban Family Welfare Services

Maternal and Child Health Services

Transport

Compensation

Mass Education

Selected program

Other services and supplies

Other expenditure

The financial requirements are as follows:

State Secretariat – Family Welfare Bureau

State Family Welfare Bureau

District Family Welfare Bureau

City Family Welfare Bureau

Area Project in Maharashtra – UNFPA – Wardha

90% Central Sponsored Scheme area project in Maharashtra – German Aided Project

World Bank Aided RCH Project

National RCH program-Nasik

RCH – Sub – Project – RTI/STI District Nasik

A pilot project with the 45 lakh population of Nasik district has been taken up. The objectives of the project are to create awareness about RTI/STI amongst general population to promote and correct treatment for RTI /STI to reduce its overall prevalence. It consists of Health Education including information on menstrual hygiene and population education for school going and out of school adolescent girls.

Area Project in RCH – Wardha

Under the Family Welfare Area Project, district Wardha has been selected from Maharashtra state for the implementation of the RCH project being assisted by the UNFPA, with the basic objectives as follows: to reduce the RTIs/STIs in the society; to reduce the maternal mortality rate; to reduce the infant mortality rate; to increase the couple protection rate.

Integrated Population and Development Project (I.P.D.) (UNFPA)

Initiated in the year 1998-2002, covering the districts of Thane, Dhule, Nandurbar, Chandrapur, Gadchiroli, Wardha and the Corporations, Thane, Pune, Kalyan, Ulhasnagar, Bhiwandi, the project is implemented by the Government of Maharashtra, through District/Corporation Societies. The project is financially assisted by the United Nations Population Fund (UNFPA) with the goals and objectives of enabling individuals and couples to achieve their personal reproductive intension and to ensure survival and development of their children through delivery of quality Reproductive and Child Health services including family planning. The activities include: training and infrastructures improvements, equipment supply, mobility support, group and communication activities, Panchayat and NGO activities, service support and project management.

Maternal and Child Health Services

Under this program the state government provides with immunization services for the pregnant mothers in terms of Tetanus, and Triple (Diptheria, Pertusis and Tetanus) vaccine for the children along with vaccination for Polio, Tuberculosis and Measles. This program has been ongoing since April 1, 1978. Since the year 1985-86 the B.C.G. vaccine is being provided for the children below one year of age. Apart from this, since the year 1986-87, the state government has been providing with Oral Rehydration Solution (ORS) for the children below five years of age in order to ensure good health for children suffering from dehydration.

Child Survival and Safe Motherhood Program

As per the state government policy, the program is initiated to provide comprehensive health care for mothers and children. The program aims at reducing the existing maternal and infant mortality rates. Special features are simple interventions for prompt referral of complicated pregnancies, timely use of ORS, identification of severe Pneumonia cases.

Mass Education

Mass Education consists of the following: showing of films, display publicity, exhibitions, monthly health magazine, posters, handbills, PVC stickers, Tin Plates, AIDS Control Program Book, Flip Charts, Jingles on Pulse Polio, AIDS and Leprosy, Flip Books, Hoardings, PVC Banners, Message Pulse Polio Card, Master cassettes-Pulse Polio, AIDS, Malaria and Leprosy, TV spots on Pulse Polio, TV Show-case, Compu-signs, Cards on Health Education, Books-Jeevan Dhara, Cinema slide, folder on health program, Poster lamination chart, audio cassettes, video cassette on health program, and health messages on wall painting.

Revised Savitri-Bai Phule Kanya Kalyan Yojana

The Government of Maharashtra has announced this scheme for the couples who have undergone sterilization operations having either one or two daughters only and no son. The main objectives of the scheme are: to improve social status of women; to give wide publicity to RCH program; to control population growths by adopting small family norms.

The Policy Statement of Maharashtra also looks at the findings of the National Family Health Survey – 2 (1998-99) and is influenced by the same, which is as follows:[6]

- Over the six-year period between NFHS-1 (1992-93) and NFHS-2 (1998-99), the average number of children per women (TFR) has declined by about half a child. Maharashtra's TFR is much lower than the current National TFR of 2.9.
- Rural women have half a child more on average than urban women.

- Women aged 15-19 accounts for 26% of total fertility. This young age of child bearing increases the health and morbidity risks for the mothers and children, and contributes to high fertility. Many women want to control their fertility
- Almost one third of married women want to stop childbearing (20%), postpone their next birth by at least two years (10%), or have already opted for sterilization (52%)
- The preferences expressed by women indicate a need for contraceptive methods to both space and limit births. Modern contraceptive use has increased since the early 1990"s. Urban use increased from 51% to 57%, while rural contraceptive use increased from 54% to 62%. Female sterilization is the most popular family planning method.
- Knowledge of the pill, IUD and condom has improved, but use of these methods (only 8% of users) remains low. These are useful for women who want to space their next birth, a preference expressed by 10 per cent of women.
- Research in low income countries has shown that spacing births by at least two years may prevent an average of one in four infant deaths.
- The picture that emerges from NFHS-2 data is one of good progress, but women still marry early having their first child soon after marriage, and use contraception only after completing their childbearing. Few contraceptive users receive essential information
- Exposure to media is moderately high. About 62% saw or heard a message on family planning during the months before the survey. Nevertheless, about 2 out of 5 women are not regularly exposed to family planning messages.
- Among women currently using contraception, few were told about other methods or side effects of their current method. This reflects a low quality of services.
- The situation is better for follow up services: about 75% of users received follow up after accepting their current method. Public medical sector remains an important source of contraceptive. 75% of users of modern contraceptives obtained

their method from the public medical sector, the same as in NFHS-1 Government sources are particularly important in rural areas (86%)

- In both urban and rural areas, the public medical sector is the main source of supply for sterilization. However, in urban areas, 28% of female sterilization occurs in the private sector, compared to only 9% in rural areas.
- Many women are still not involved in personal health care decisions, only half of women report having a voice in decision about their own health, younger women are much more less likely than older women to participate in decisions about their own health care. Urban, non-slum women, and women with a middle school or higher education are more likely to be involved in decisions regarding their health care. Maternal health services improve.
- 90 per cent of mothers received at-least one ante-natal check up from 1992 (85% of births), 75 per cent of mothers received 2 or more doses of tetanus toxoid vaccine, slightly up from NFHS-1, 85 per cent of mothers received iron folic acid supplementation. Of those, only 84 per cent received the recommended 3 month course.
- Professional assistance at delivery increased to 60%in NFHS-2
- Women's nutritional status is poor, about two-fifths of women are malnourished, with a BMI below 18.5 kg/m, nearly one third of pregnant women have moderate to severe Anemia, compared to non pregnant women.
- Infant mortality declined from 58 deaths per 1000 birth during 1984-1988 to 44 deaths in 1994-1998, an average rate of decline of 1.4 infant deaths per 1000 live births per year. Maharashtra has the seventh lowest infant mortality rate in the country. However despite the decline one of every 23rd infant before age one & one in 17 die before age 5. The infant mortality is 55% higher among children born to mothers under age 20, than among children born to mothers age 20-29
- Immunization coverage high, between NFHS-1 & NFSH-2, proportion of children who received no immunization dropped

from 8%-2%. The proportion of children who received at least one vaccine is nearly 98n% while 78% are fully immunized. Despite high rates, more than one in three of illiterate mothers & children belonging to schedule tribes are not fully immunized.

- Many children are Anaemic; overall three-fourths of children under age three are Anaemic. Most of these children suffer from mild or moderate Anaemia. Anaemic children are at greater risk of infection, impaired mental skills, physical development and poor school performance.
- Malnutrition levels remain high. Half of children under age three suffer from low weight for age-also called as under weight, a measure of both short and long term under nutrition. The same proportion are undernourished to the extent their growth has been stunted, they suffer from low height-for-age (40%). About one in five children have both low height and low weight, also called as Wasting. Wasting is associated with a failure to receive adequate nutrition in the period immediately before the survey and may be the result of seasonal variations in food supply or recent episodes of illness. The percentage of under weight children has remained unchanged since the early 1990s
- Poor feeding practices begin in infancy. Only about two in five infants under four months are exclusively breastfed, and only 31% of those aged 6-9 months are being fed solid and mushy foods. Starting supplements at 6 month is critical for meeting Protein, Energy and micronutrient needs.

Policy Changes in Maharashtra-Components of RCH Program Stated by the Center

- Women's health, safe motherhood (including safe management of unwanted pregnancy and abortion
- Women's development
- Child Health (child survival and child development)
- Adolescent Health (sexuality development, adolescence education and vocational component)

- Effective Family Planning (Ensuring Informed choice, Counselling, gender equality and greater male participation)
- Prevention, detection and management of Reproductive Tract Infections, Sexually Transmitted Infections, HIV/AIDS and cancer of the reproductive system.
- Prevention and management of infertility and other reproductive disorders
- Prevention, detection and management of genetic and environmental disorders
- Reproductive health care of elderly persons

Table 5.5

State declared its 'Population Policy' on 8th March 2000

Following Goals have been set to be achieved by the year 2004

Indicator	*Present Status (SRS)*	*Goal*	
Birth Rate	Maharashtra	2004	2010
	21.1(1999)	18	15
Death rate	7.5(1999)	6.4	5
Total Fertility Rate	2.5(1999)	2.1	1.8
Infant Mortality Rate	48(1999)	25	15
Neonatal Mortality Rate	35	20	10

Source: ***Health Status, 2002*** **(Public Health Department, Government of Maharashtra).**

To achieve the above Goals Special emphasis on the following is laid down in the policy statement:

- To improve Reproductive and Child Health Program management by strengthening, monitoring and supervision.
- To enhance Accessibility, Availability and Acceptability of quality services to meet the Unmet Needs.
- To ensure better utilization of the services by increasing awareness among the community about the available facilities and also about the factors affecting demographic processes like age at marriage, son preference, safe motherhood practices and new born care.

- To organize special health service camps and Adolescent Clinics.
- To involve related Departments and Non-Government Organizations (NGO) Community Based Organization (CBO) and Local Self Governments in the program.

The Health Schemes implemented by Government of Maharashtra exclusively with regards to RCH are as follows:

1. Establishment of First Referral Units. (F.R.U.)

There are 350 Rural Hospitals in the state. Out of these, 123 have been considered for establishing as First Referral Units (F.R.U.) All the F.R.Us have been supplied with Kits E to P. To operationalize the F.R.U.s- Posts of Specialist (Gynaecologist/Surgeon, "Paediatrician or Physician" & Anaesthetist) have been created at every FRU. All F.R.Us have been provided with Rs. 10.00 Lakh for repairs and renovation of labour Room & Operation Theatre, upgrading water supply and electrification, Provision for using services of Gynaecologist, & Anaesthetist on contract basis.

2. 24-Hour Delivery Scheme

Table 5.6

The scheme is implemented in following four districts in the State

Sr. No.	*District*	*No. of PHCs*
1.	Nanded	53
2.	Parbhani	47
3.	Jalna	28
4.	Yavatmal	57
	Total	**185**

The scheme is implemented to encourage institutional deliveries in order to reduce maternal and infant mortality. There is good response and increase in the number of institutional deliveries is observed. The Medical Officers, Nurses and Attendants are given incentive under this scheme.

3. Appointment of Consultants

It is proposed to appoint Consultants in following areas on contractual basis, at state level: (i) Finance (ii) Cold chain (iii) Monitoring and evaluation (iv) Promotion of contraceptives (v) IEC

4. RCH Camps

In order to have an easy access for the treatment of RTI/STI, Disease Diagnostic Camps are proposed under the scheme. Following type of services are provided in the camp: Information counseling and services; Contraceptive methods; Menstrual regulation; MTP services; Gynaecological problems (RTI/STI); and Adolescent problems.

5. Establishment of Neonatal Care Unit

In order to bring down the Infant Mortality Rate from 48/1000 live birth to 25 by 2004, it is essential to improve the Neonatal Care. It is, therefore, proposed to establish Neonatal Care Units in following districts. Ratnagiri, Osmanabad, Sangli, Wardha, Sindhudurg, Buldhana, Solapur, Raigad, Satara, Ahmednagar, Beed and Bhandara. The state government has already sanctioned Neonatal Intensive Care Units at Jalgaon, Parbhani, Kolhapur, Akola and Latur. Supply of essential equipments in the Delivery Room, Ambulance facility to transport low birth weight babies and supply of instruments for ICU are also included.

6. Referral Transport

It is observed that for maternal death, the unavailability of transport is one reason. Therefore, under the scheme, it is proposed to place Rs. 5,000/- with the local gram panchayat for first year and Rs. 4000/- Rs. 3000/- Rs. 2000/- Rs. 1000/- subsequently. The scheme is to be implemented in selected 50 villages of 10 districts viz. Nanded, Nandurbar, Dhule, Solapur, Parbhani, Bhandara, Gadchiroli, Aurangabad, Jalna and Osmanabad. Beneficiary will get Rs. 300/- for transport.

7. Utilization of Services of Private Gynecologist and Anaesthetist on Contract Basis

In order to provide emergency obstetric services, the Specialist are required. They are not available at many of the First Referral

Units. Therefore, a provision has been made to utilize the services of private Gynecologists and Anaesthetist by paying them consultation charges.

8. Training of Dais

In number of villages, the delivery is conducted by the Traditional Birth Attendants. In order to reduce Maternal Mortality and Infant Mortality safe delivery practices are essential. Under the scheme, The Dais, who are conducting the deliveries will be trained at selected FRUs and also required Orientation Training will be given.

9. NGO Involvement

The Government of India has selected four mother NGOs in the state. These NGOs are working since 1998-99. They have so far registered 110 Field NGOs from the districts assigned to them.

Table 5.7

Mother NGO	*No. of Field NGOs*	*Districts allotted*
Society of Services to Voluntary Agencies (SOSVA)	37	Pune, Nagpur, Ahmednagar, Raigad, Mumbai, Amravati,Latur, Nanded, Wardha, Gadchiroli Chandrapur, Yavatmal, Buldhana, Akola Washim, Osmanabad, Satara Bhandara, Gondia.
Sevadham Trust, Pune	30	Sindhudurg, Solapur, Thane Kolhapur, Ratnagiri, Parabhani Sangli, Hingoli
Pravara Medical Trust, Loni	26	Beed, Aurangabad, Jalna Dist. Ahmednagar
Godavari Foundation, Jalgaon.	17	Nasik, Dhule, Nandurbar, Jalgaon, Buldhana, Yavatmal

Source: ***Health Status, 2002*** **(Public Health Department, Government of Maharashtra).**

The Family Welfare Program of the State Government Comprises of the following: Sterilization

The sterilization program is well established in the state. There are operating facilities available for sustained programme. In the year 2000-2001, 109% sterilizations were performed against the Expected level of achievement. The high light of the performance is that 40% sterilizations were performed on two issues. This indicates quality of the programme and the acceptability by the Community. The performance is mainly through Female Sterilization operations. The Population Policy is now giving stress on Male sterilizations. Therefore, a special scheme promoting *No Scalpel Vasectomy (NSV)* is being implemented. Under the scheme, the Medical Officers have been trained and NSV camps are organized.

Urban Family Welfare Program

The 2001 Census has registered the urban population of 42%. To implement the Health Programmes in the urban are, proper Health Infrastructure is not available. The Urban Family Welfare Centres and Urban Health Posts have been established as follows:

Table 5.8

Sr. No.	*Type of Institutions*	*Govt.*	*Local Bodiestal*	*Vol. Organs*	*To*
	URBAN FAMILY WELFARE CENTRES				
1.	Type-I	10	12	0	22
	Type-II	0	9	1	10
	Type-III	10	15	17	42
	Total	20	36	18	74
	URBAN HEALTH POSTS				
2.	Type-A	3	9	0	12
	Type-B	2	14	0	16
	Type-C	9	31	2	42
	Type-D	25	155	30	210
	Total	**39**	**209**	**32**	**280**

Source: ***Health Status*, 2002 (Public Health Department, Government of Maharashtra).**

The abovementioned centers and the staff receive 100% grants from Government of India through State Government. The targets are allotted to the institution for sterilization performance. The performance is monitored and the work of the Centre is evaluated.

3. Post Partum Program

The Post Partum Programme is Maternity center based Family Welfare Program. There are five type of centers recognized on the basis of the workload of obstetric cases, abortion and MTP cases. The acceptors of performance are direct and indirect. The institutions are expected to complete the target of sterilization, Cu-T. On the basis of this, the grants are released. In the state, following Post Partum Centers are sanctioned.

Table 5.9

Sr. No.	*Agency*	*No. of Post Partum Centers*					
		A-Teach	*A- Non-Teach*	*B Type*	*C Type*	*Sub District*	*Total*
1.	Govt.	8	7	7	14	47	83
2.	Local Body	3	2	3	1	12	21
3.	Vol. Orgn.	1	2	1	3	10	17
	Total	**12**	**11**	**11**	**18**	**69**	**121**

Source: ***Health Status, 2002*** **(Public Health Department, Government of Maharashtra).**

4. Award Scheme

In order to motivate the Health Staff, an Award Scheme offering Cash incentive has been started from August 2000. The Award Scheme is for Medical Officers, ANMs and also for Panchayat Samitis. The Selection Committee of District Collector, CEO, ZP, DHO and District RCH Officer will select the Health Staff for the Award.

5. Revised Savitribai Phule Kanya Kalyan Yojana:

The scheme is revised from 1st May 2000 and is applicable for:

(i) Couples below poverty line.

(ii) Couples accepting sterilization with only one daughter and no son, will receive Rs. 10,000/- as Fixed Deposit in the daughter's name, which the daughter will receive it after completing 18 years. An additional amount of Rs. 5,000/- will be awarded as a Five Year Fixed Deposit for the girl completing 10th Standard, provided she does not get marry before the age of 20 years.

(iii) Similar scheme is applicable for couples with two daughters and no son. The amount is Rs. 5,000/- per daughter.

6. Monitoring of Age at Marriage:

(i) Anti-Early Marriage Fortnight.

(ii) Gathering of Newly married couples.

(iii) Reporting of marriages before the age of 18.

(iv) Monthly Early Marriage (EM) reports.

7. Prevention of misuse of Pre-Natal Sex Determination Act (PNDT Act)

The Act came in to force on 1st January 1996. The objective is to regulate the activity of the Genetic Counselling Centers, Genetic Laboratories and Genetic Clinics. The facility is expected to be used for detecting Genetic disorders. However, it was observed that the facility has been mis-utilized by getting the Foetus aborted after it is diagnosed as a female. This has resulted in to the imbalance between Sex Ratio. The 2001 Census data reveals that the sex ratio for male/ female in Maharashtra State has come down to 922 compared to 934 in the 1991 census. The Supreme Court has already directed all the States to take stringent measures against the mis-utilization of the act. In view of this, the State has already taken following actions.

- State Appropriate Authority is the Additional Director of Health Services (FW), Pune
- Advisory Committee Appointed.
- District Appropriate Authorities appointed
- Registration of the equipment has been made compulsory for all the centers.
- Information, Education & Communication Campaign for community awareness regarding the provisions of the Act and punishment for violation of rule has been undertaken on large scale. A regular review is taken at the Govt. level.

8. School Health

The health check up of the School going children will timely correct the defects in the early stages and will result in proper physical and mental development of the child. In order that this is done in the primary stage School Health Check-ups are organized since last five years on campaign basis. The examination of the students in Class I to IV Standard takes place in October, November every year. The data collected indicate that the activity is useful. The cases identified are referred to the Health Institution where proper treatment, surgical intervention is carried out.

9. Immunization Program

The Universal Immunization against vaccine preventable diseases such as Tuberculosis, Polio, Diphtheria, Pertusis, Tetanus and Measles is routinely carried out. The routine Immunization Programme has received very good response from the community.

10. Polio Eradication

The success of the Immunization against Polio has laid to the strategy of Polio Eradication. The Government of India undertook the activity of Pulse Polio Immunization since last five years. The IEC activities and excellent implementation plan has resulted into 98 to 99% coverage and reduction in the polio cases. Through the support from WHO for AFP Surveillance, the programme is being monitored efficiently. The Community response as well as NGO involvement and the commitment of the State Government has resulted in nearing the Polio eradication final stage. The strategy of the program consists of: Strengthening routine immunization program; Organization of National Immunization Days; Organization of Intensive Pulse Polio Immunization; Effective AFP Surveillance.

11. Training under RCH Program[7]

The Government of India has identified National Institute of Health & Family Welfare (NIHFW) as the Nodal Agency for Training activities under the RCH Programme. The State has formed the "State Level RCH Training Co-Ordination Committee". According to the guidelines of NIHFW and in consultation with the Collaborating

Training Institute (CTI) i.e. KEM Hospital & Research Centre, Pune, the Comprehensive Training Action Plan (CTP) has been prepared. Following type of training activities are under progress:

(a) *Integrated Skill Development Training (ISDT) for M.O., LHV, ANM (12 days):* The Training is Hospital based. The objective is to improve the skills of the workers for improving the quality of Service delivery.

(b) *Integrated Skill Development Training (ISDT):* For Male Health Supervisor and Workers (6 days). The objective is to involve the Male Health Supervisor and Workers in the RCH Program activities.

(c) *Specialized Skill Development Training (SST) (12 days):* The Medical Officers are sent for Training in Mini lap, Laparoscopic sterilization, Medical Termination of Pregnancy (MTP) and No Scalpel Vasectomy (NSV). The ANMs and LHVs are trained in Intra Uterine Device (Cu-T) insertion Technique. The objective is to increase the trained and skilled manpower, so that, the performance will improve in quantity as well as in quality.

(d) *Management Training (1 week):* The Institute of Health Management, Pachod, District Aurangabad has been identified for the training of State/Regional and district level Officers.

(e) *Communication (11 Days):* Public Health Institute, Nagpur and HFWTC, Pune have been identified for the training of Health supervisors.

Financial Provisions and Expenditure

The financial provisions for the Reproductive Health programs in the State are made from various sources as follows:

- Central government funds
- State government funds
- Foreign funding agencies like GTZ, UNFPA, and development sections of various embassies
- World Bank

The ongoing RCH project being implemented since 1997 is aided by the World Bank. Following has been the fund flow since its inception.

Table 5.10

Year	*Reference*	*Rs. In lakhs*	*Remarks*
1997-98	Form GFR 19-A No.M12015/1/97.FWB(I) Dated February 9, 98.	150.00	Additional installment
1997-98	Form GFR 19-A No.M12015/1/97.FWB(I) Dated March 25, 98.	75.00	National Component
1997-98	Form GFR 19-A No.M12015/1/97.FWB(I) Dated March 31, 98	215.00	National Component
1997-98	Form GFR 19-A No.M12015/1/97.FWB(I) Dated March 31, 1998	132.84	Additional installment
1997-98	Form GFR 19-A No.M12015/1/97.FWB(I) Dated March 31, 1998	75.00	Sub-project
1997-98	Form GFR 19-A No.G.25020/1/97.RCH(DC) Dated April 29, 98.	3.51	MCH registered
1998-99	Form GFR 19-A No.M.12015/1/98.FWB(I) Dated April 27, 98	41.63	1st installment
1998-99	Form GFR 19-A No.M.12015/1/98.FWB(I) Dated October 21, 98	1.39	3rd installment
1998-99	Form GFR 19-A No.M.12015/1/98.FWB(I) Dated October 20, 98	154.08	4th installment
1998-99	Form GFR 19-A No.M.12015/1/98.FWB(I) Dated March 31, 99	7.44	Zillah Saksharta Samiti (ZSS) funds
1998-99	Form GFR 19-A No.M.12015/2/98.MCH Dated August 19, 98	33.30	Allocation
1998-99	Form GFR 19-A No.G.20011/1/98.CH/PI Dated November 17, 98	79.00	

(Contd...)

Year	Reference	Rs. In lakhs	Remarks
1999-2000	Form GFR 19-A No.M.12015/1/99 FWB(I) Dated June 30, 99	5.13	ZSS
1999-2000	Form GFR 19-A No.M.12015/1/99 FWB(I) Dated Aug 24, 99	13.10	Cold chain
1999-2000	Form GFR 19-A No.M.12015/1/99 FWB (I)Dated Nov 11, 99	3.19	ZSS
1999-2000	Form GFR 19-A No.L.25012/9/99 FWB(I) Dated May 10, 99	10.27	ZSS – IEC activities – Latur Chandrapur and Bhandara
2000-2001	Form GFR 19-A No.M.12015/1/2000 FWB(I) Dated Februray 20, 2001	165.4	Civil works (additional installment)
2000-2001	Form GFR 19-A No.M.12015/1/2001 FWB(I) Dated December 18, 2000	36.58	Cold chain (additional installment)
2001-2002	Form GFR 19-A No.M.12015/1/2001 FWB(I) Dated September 5, 2001	36.78	Cold chain
2001-2002	Form GFR 19-A No.M.12015/1/2001 FWB(I) Dated November 11, 2001	364.46	Civil works (additional installment)
2001-2002	Form GFR 19-A No.M.12015/1/2001 FWB(I) Dated October 22, 2001	176.08	Dai training and RCH component

Source: **The abovementioned financial data has been procured from the Additional Director, Family Welfare Bureau, Pune.**

Information, Education and Communication efforts and programs undertaken by the State IEC Bureau

Introduction

Health Education is an integral part of each and every health program. The Maharashtra state health directory describes the work of State Information Education and Communication (IEC) Bureau as cement, which binds together the bricks of a wall. State Health

Education Bureau was established for undertaking the following activities. In the year 1996, this bureau was renamed as State Information Education and Communication Bureau. Its tasks include:[8]

- To monitor health education activities conducted at district level.
- To procure, distribute and monitor the health education material and equipment.
- To undertake field education studies.
- To publish monthly health Bulletin (Arogya Patrika) for continuing education of health personnel.
- To celebrate World Health Day and other days related to important Health themes.
- To design and bring out educational aids for health personnel and masses.

In the last few years the bureau has produced and supplied a number of Health Education material such as exhibition sets, audio visual equipments, slide sets, audio visual equipments, slide sets, films, booklets, folders, posters, tin plates to the districts and also explored the new media for publicity such as painting on S.T. buses and display of hoardings in prominent places.

Implementation Mechanisms of IEC Program

Following is the existing system of the implementation of IEC program.

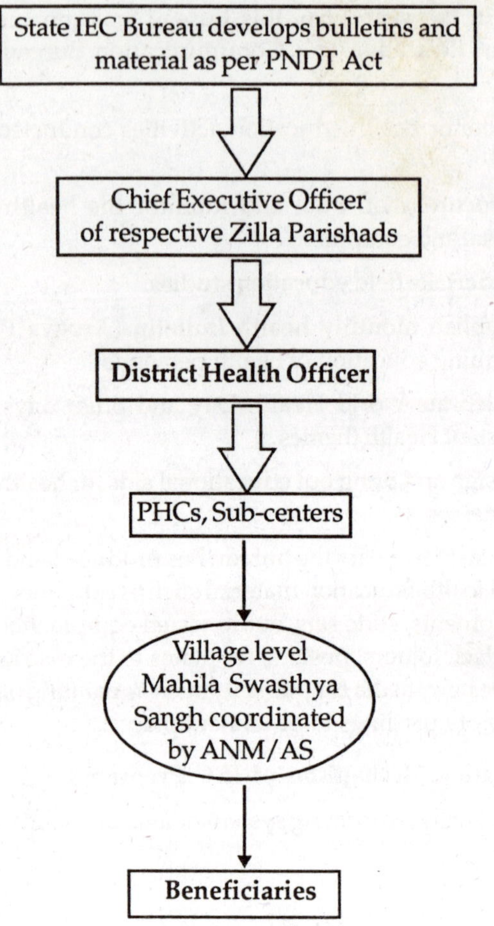

Diagram No. 5.1

Process of Material preparation and development

With regards to the material preparation by the IEC bureau the following steps are followed:

- Organization of the workshop for the artists, District Education and Media Officers (DEMOs), photographers of all the districts.

- Introduction of the theme and the concept of the topic for which the material is to be prepared.
- Discussion of ideas on first two days of the workshop.
- Prepare rough sketches, ideas, slogans and posters for the same.
- Extension of guidance for the same from the resource person.
- Preparation of the draft.
- Pre-testing in the villages to estimate the understanding and grasping of the people as well as the viability and the capacity of the material prepared.

With the abovementioned steps, the IEC material for the purpose of distribution and dissemination is prepared and developed in a very democratic and professional manner. Apart from this some material and some messages are also extended to the bureau from central government or other governmental and non governmental funding agencies.

IEC Budget Under Public Health Department

The Performance Budget (Part I)[9] of the Public Health Department lists out the IEC section in collaboration with the Department of Nutrition, and hence the programs are undertaken jointly.

The budget classification both activity-wise and object-wise is in two parts viz. Nutritional Education and Bureau of Health Education comprising of mainly salaries, travel expenses, office expenses, motor vehicles, materials and supplies, diet charges and other charges. The financial availability is made from the Budget Head 2211 of the department.

IEC Budget of Family Welfare Component of Public Health Department

As stated in the Performance Budget (Part II) [10] 'Family Welfare', of the Public Health Department of the Maharashtra state, the subject head used for the IEC activities is Mass Education and Publicity, which includes Orientation Training Camps in all Districts, Corporations and other Institutions for motivating the people and to achieve that aim of Family Welfare Program. Para-media such as exhibitions, film shows, cinema-slides, songs and dramas etc, through which the Family Welfare Centers acquaint rural population with importance and the methods of Family Welfare and Planned Parenthood. Similarly, exhibitions are also conducted at the Urban Family Welfare Centers.

The overall performance under this budget head include:

1. Planning of Health Education and Family Welfare publicity program.
2. Production of Health Education material and provide it at the regional level.
3. To arrange exhibitions of Health.
4. To involve in Health Education (population education to Mahila Swasthya Sangh & Youth Forums.)
5. To publish and distribute the health magazine through out the state in every month.
6. To make evaluation of Health Education media and type of media.
7. To manage the Health Education program as per Index.
8. To increase the various type of Health Education and Family Welfare program by using the media and publicity: a) Film Show; b) Health Exhibition; c) Block meetings.
9. To take review of Health Education in the State.
10. To celebrate the World Health day, World Population day etc.

The Performance Budget states the financial requirements in Budget Head 2210 of the department with regards to the activity Classification, which comprises of: Mass Education; World Bank Aided Project in Health Education; Bilateral assistance from UK Government for Health Education. The object-wise classification of the same is further divided into the office expenses, advertising and sales publicity.

An Overview of IEC Activities Undertaken in the State in Last Three Years

This section describes the production and distribution of monthly health magazines, poster, handbills, P.V.C. stickers, tin plates, AIDS control program book, Flip charts, jingles on pulse polio-AIDS-Leprosy, flip books, hoardings, P.V.C banners, message pulse polio card, master cassettes, T.V. spots, T.V. Show case, compu-signs, cards on health education, jivandhara, cinema slide, folders, poster lamination charts, audio cassettes, video cassettes, and wall paintings in the state in the last three years.

The state IEC Bureau has produced a lot of important IEC material, which is related to various health issues and especially focusing upon the gender equality, misuse of PNDT act, sanitation and hygiene and the importance to be given to maternal and child health. Within the material preparation the focus is more on the print material as compared to the electrical and electronic media. However, some very good educational documentary films like Dai Ma, Importance of Breast-feeding, *Don Aapatyavar Shastrakriya* (operation after two children), *Swayamvar, Shevantacha lagin, Diwas Tujhe Phulayache, Vay Wadhtana,* mainly focusing upon adolescent reproductive health and general care during pregnancy are produced in the Marathi language.

The Personnel Summary of the State IEC Bureau

The State IEC Bureau comprises of the following officials from both medical and non-medical background:

1. Joint Director of Health Services (Cl-I) (Medical);
2. Deputy Director of Health Services (Cl-I) (Non – Medical);
3. Assistant Director of Health Services (Cl-II) (Medical);
4. Health Education Officer (Cl-II) (Non Medical);
5. Office Superintendent (Cl. III);
6. Assistant Superintendent (Cl. III);
7. Statistician (Cl. III);
8. Assistant Librarian (Cl. III);
9. Health Propogandist (Cl. III);
10. Artist – cum – Photographer (Cl. III);
11. Steno Typist (Cl. III);
12. Senior Clerk (Cl. III);

13. Junior Clerk (Cl. III);
14. Driver (Cl. III);
15. Driver – cum – projectionist (Cl. III);
16. Projectionist (Cl. III).

The Class IV employees comprise of Peons, Majdoor, Cleaner, Night watchman, Packer and Sweeper.

The Personnel Summary of the District IEC Unit

District Education and Media Officers (DEMO)	–	1
Artist	–	1
Projectionist	–	1
Driver	–	1
Health assistant	–	1
Peon	–	1

Management Information System (MIS)

The MIS of the state IEC bureau is as follows:

The reporting of progress of previous month at block level is done on 1st to 3rd of every month. During this time the information is collected and compiled by the PHC from the field level that is sub-centers, extended to the block level, further consolidated at the block level and is forwarded to the district head quarters. The reporting and compilation of the collected information is done by the DHO between 3rd and 5th of every month. This is further forwarded to the Deputy Director of Health Services (DDHS) – Circle office – (DDHS-Akola is the circle office in case of Amravati district. In Maharashtra totally there are 8 such circle offices, that is Pune, Thane, Nasik, Akola, Nagpur, Latur, Kolhapur, and Aurangabad) and here the total compilation is done between 5th and 8th of every month. The DDHS forwards the reports to the Additional Director, Family Welfare Bureau, Pune and here the entire information is compiled district wise as against the set indicators and forwarded to the Director General of Health Services (DGHS) Mumbai. The information at the DGHS level are reviewed and sent to the Secretary – Public Health Department.

Monitoring and Inspection System

The Health Education Officer (HEO) of the State IEC Bureau, Pune, is responsible for the monitoring and has to pay field visits to different districts for ten days of every month. In the inspection visits, the HEO inspects the proper distribution of the material to the sub-centers, the display of the material distribution and the utilization of the same at the field level.

An Overview of IEC Activities Undertaken in Amravati District in Last Three Years

As stated in the performance budget –2002-2003 of the Public Health Department, following activities have been undertaken in Amravati district:

Table 5.11

Year	*No. of Film Shows*	*No. of display publicity*	*Exhibitions*
2000-2001	185	10,000	245
2001-2002	140	5,000	42
2002-2003	200	10,000	260

Special Efforts by the IEC Unit of Melghat Region in Amrawati District

Special efforts by the IEC unit of Amravati DHO office have been undertaken in last few years. These efforts have concentrated on programs and inputs in the Dharni and Chikhaldara blocks of Melghat region. Following are the initiatives taken:

- Folk songs in Korku language giving messages on immunization, small family, sanitation and child health transmitted on All India Radio
- Relaying documentary films like *Prayashchit, Kusumche Lagin, Man Gaye Ustad, and Pate ki Baat* – fosusing on the malnutrition issue and maternal and child health on the local city cable channel through Zilla Parishad.
- Writing of health messages on trees, stones on the roadside and rivers in Korku language to help them eradicate superstitions.

- Celebration of nutrition week and lectures and film shows in the community settings of the tribal villages.
- Special video and audio cassettes with songs and dances providing messages of immunization to the community.
- Special audio cassettes based on religious songs of the local goddesses – based on the messages of health.
- Special exhibitions on health care.
- Specially designed street plays giving messages and information regarding AIDS.

Public Health Schemes Implemented by the Maharashtra State Government: ***With Special Reference to the Melghat Region of Amravati District***

The Public Health Department has been implementing special schemes in the Melghat region of Amravati district since the year 1995-96. The Melghat region covers two tribal blocks of Dharni and Chikhaldara. The special schemes are implemented in these blocks as a result of the policy changes emerging from the aftermath of the Infant Mortality Crisis in the year 1993. The crisis was said to have resulted due to malnutrition amongst the infants in the area. Over a period of years a number of schemes have been designed and implemented and have gradually being termed as "Melghat Pattern", which is now being replicated in the other tribal districts of Maharashtra.

The Melghat pattern comprises of the following schemes[11]:

1. Nav Sanjeevan Yojana

The State Government has selected the district having tribal population for the implementation of Special Programs. In following districts, Nav Sanjeevan Yojana has been introduced in the following districts:

1 Thane

2. Raigad

3. Nasik

4. Dhule

5. Jalgaon
6. Ahmednagar
7. Nandurbar
8. Amravati
9. Yavatmal
10. Nanded
11. Nagpur
12. Pune
13. Gondia
14. Chandrapur
15. Gadchiroli

Following activities are implemented:

- Pre-monsoon health check-ups of Tribal mothers and children and treatment
- Regular water quality monitoring
- Filling of vacancies
- Monthly Examination of Grade III and Grade IV children
- Facility of diet to patient and one relative at PHC and RH
- Maintaining the mobility of the vehicles
- Ensuring availability of Drugs for epidemic control at the Health Institutions

2. Integrated Tribal Development Project (ITDP)

Following tribal districts are covered:

1. Thane
2. Nasik
3. Nandurbar
4. Amravati
5. Gadchiroli.

The schemes implemented through the special action plans with regards to Reproductive and Child Health are:

1. Matrutwa Anudan Yojana

The schemes are implemented through out the year. The beneficiary is the pregnant mother. Rs. 400/- are given to the beneficiary. The objective is to support the diet and encouraging the beneficiary to accept safe motherhood concept.

2. Flying Squads for the Inspection of Work

The flying squad has been appointed by the Directorate of Health Services, Mumbai in order to inspect the work being done by the officials in the Melghat blocks.

3. Dai Training

The Dais conducting the delivery are called for quarterly one day orientation training. They are paid Rs. 40/- as honorarium and Rs. 10/- as meeting expenses. The Dais are oriented about safe delivery practices and new born care.

4. Pada Swayamsevak Scheme

The scheme is implemented from May to December every year. The Pada worker is paid Rs. 300/- per month. 5530 posts of Pada Workers have been sanctioned. They are expected to perform following activities:

1. Water disinfection.
2. Tablet Chloroquine distribution to fever patients.
3. ORS packets to diarrhoea patients.
4. Information of epidemic outbreak to PHC.
5. Assistance in the distribution of supplementary diet.

5. Deputation of Pediatricians during the Epidemic Prone Period

The pediatricians are deputed by the Directorate of Health Services during the monsoons, which is the epidemic prone period, in order to provide with immediate and instant services to the people.

6. Appointment of Honorary Doctors

The scheme is implemented from June to December. The appointed Doctor is paid Rs. 6000/- per month. 132 posts have been sanctioned. The Doctor is expected to carry out the following duties:

- Health check-ups of mothers and children in every Pada/ village in the area.
- Treatment of mothers and children having health problems
- Examination of children in Anganwadi.

Table 5.12

Honorary Doctors & Pada Swayamsevak

District	*Honorary Doctors*		*Pada Swayansevak*	
	Sanctioned	*Filled in*	*Sanctioned*	*Filled in*
Thane	35	35	1872	1872
Nasik	25	25	968	968
Nandurbar	265	25	1312	1279
Gadchiroli	22	25	239	239
Amravati	25	25	1139	1139
Total	**132**	**132**	**5530**	**5497**

Source: ***Health Status, 2002*** **(Public Health Department, Government of Maharashtra).**

7. Establishment of Paediatric Intensive Care Unit

The Intensive Care Unit has been sanctioned as a permanent scheme for Dharni and Chikhaldara Rural Hospitals. Following provisions have been made:

- Five posts of staff Nurses sanctioned.
- One room of the R.H. converted in to Warm Room.
- Care of Low Birth Weight Babies.
- Use of Thermo-Cole Boxes.

8. Compensation for Loss of Wages to Either Parent of the Grade III and Grade IV Children Admitted for Treatment

- 26 Talukas of 5 districts have been included.
- Rs. 14/- per day per child can be spent on the treatment.
- Arrangement for residence of the parents.

(The Government Resolutions (GRs) related to the abovementioned schemes of Melghat pattern are enclosed as annexure)

Reporting System

The responsibility of reporting on the status and performance of the abovementioned schemes lies with the Assistant Director of Health Services (Tribal areas) stationed in the Directorate of Health Services, Mumbai. The reporting is done on a monthly basis with the following nine sub-heads.

Institution status in ITDP and Nav Sanjeevan area

Manpower and vacancy position

Vehicle status

Water disinfection status

Malnutrition children status

Medical examination of anganwadi children

Infant mortality

Matrutwa Anudan Yojana

Dai meetings

This process of reporting system ensures the review of the work being done in every month.

REFERENCES

1. Government of India, *National Population Policy 2000*, (New Delhi, India, Department of Family Welfare, Govt. of India, 2000).

2. Nalini Paranjpe, *Impact of Various Schemes Related to Elementary Education: A Comparative Study of Girls Literacy in Maharashtra and Madhya Pradesh* (Project sponsored by the Planning Commission, Government of India, 2000), pp.19-21.

3. *State Health Directory, 1994*, (Department of Public Health, Government of Maharashtra).

4. Government of Maharashtra, *Performance Budget* – Public Health Department, 2002-2003.

5. Data taken from *Performance Budget, 2002-2003 Part I*, (Public Health Department, Government of Maharashtra).

6. *National Family Health Survey, 1998-99*, (Mumbai, International Institute of Population Sciences).

7. *Health Status, 2002* (Public Health Department, Government of Maharashtra).

8. Government of Maharashtra, Health Directory Maharashtra – 1994, Mumbai, 1994 p. 256.
9. Data taken from *Performance Budget, 2002-2003 Part-I*, n. 5.
10. Data taken from *Performance Budget, 2002-2003 Part – II* (Public Health Department, Family Welfare, Government of Maharashtra).
11. *Health Status, 2002* (Public Health Department, Government of Maharashtra).

6

NGOs and Policy Implementation

Introduction

Nongovernmental Organizations and Voluntary Organizations are a key component of civil society in a democratic policy. They play an important role as parallel agencies that contribute to the making of public policy. The social sector in particular has seen a remarkable activity of such organizations. This chapter therefore looks into the role played by such organizations in structuring and implementing policy.

Selected Efforts Made by Various Nongovernmental Organizations (NGOs) in Advocacy at Policy and Implementation Levels

Though we have seen that the advocacy work and research in the field of reproductive health has its roots in the work of Dr. R. D. Karve in the year 1929, it is equally important to have a look at a number of efforts being undertaken by various organizations, that is voluntary organizations, pressure groups, universities and research bodies in the field of policy making and policy implementation.

Various Non-Governmental Organizations (NGOs) working in the field of Reproductive Health have contributed to the policy making and policy implementation process associated with Reproductive Health activities. Accordingly, the efforts undertaken by the NGOs in Maharashtra have been quoted here:

Ashish Gram Rachna Trust, an NGO working in the District Aurangabad has been involved in community health programs since 1977. The basic component was training of TBAs in maternal and child health, selecting and training female community health workers and establishing health posts to provide medical services at village level. These interventions cover 50 villages of Paithan block in the district. Apart from this the organization is involved in Health Education programs for the adolescents between the age group of 9 & 16 years.

Bharat Agro Industries Foundation (BAIF), established in 1967, has been working in the field of community health in Pune district. BAIF overtly recognized the congruence and linkages between health and livelihood programs to improve nutrition sanitation and water as critical aspects for improving community health. The organization operates women's clinic in two villages, focusing mainly on RTI, STI and other gynaecological problems. It is also involved in research activities with regards to gynecological morbidity, perception of women's health and attitude regarding reproductive health.

King Edward Memorial (KEM) Hospital, a leading charitable trust in Pune was established in 1912 and is associated with BJ Medical College for under graduate and post-graduate students as teaching institution. It offers a constellation of reproductive health services and is involved in research activities since 1973. One of the most important research work undertaken by the institution is about adolescent sexuality and fertility. The specific objective of the study were to identify adolescent knowledge, attitudes and practices regarding sex, fertility, contraception, RTI, STI, and gender differences in the dynamics of decision making at the house hold level on matter related to sexual behaviour.

Mahatma Gandhi Institute of Medical Sciences (MGIMS), Wardha, established in 1944, became the first hospital to train ANMs, in the year 1945. The reproductive interventions began with the project in 19 villages in the year 1987. Reproductive health is a part of community health package though this is largely limited to maternal and child-care. The main objective of the project is to reduce maternal and infant mortality, and morbidity within this framework. An innovative reproductive health project at the hospital level is being implemented for the unwed mothers and their babies with the objective to prevent women from resorting to illegal or unhealthy abortion practices due to socio-culture pressures.

Navjeet Community Health Center, Mumbai, established in the year 1979 is involved in reproductive health care in the slums of Mumbai. Mainly grass root workers supported by weekly clinics held at the center provide health care at the community level. The reproductive health problems like menstrual problems, RTI, STI, are treated at hospital level on an ad-hoc basis as and when patient comes.

Society for Education Action and Research in Community Health (SEARCH), established in Gadchiroli district by Dr. Abhay Bang and Dr. Rani Bang one of the least developed districts in Maharashtra are accredited with innovative interventions in the area of reproductive health since 1986. An action research study in the year 1989 found that 92% of women from the selected sample had one or more gynecological diseases with an average of 3.6 gynaecological problems per women. The study became a landmark and resulted in to rigorous activities in reproductive health and caters to health education through traditional birth attendance, and special inputs regarding both male and female reproductive health as well as adolescent reproductive health.

Center for Enquiry into Health and Allied Themes (CEHAT)[1], a registered organization works as a research based think tank and advocacy group to advocate on the issues related to primary health care in the country. With its administrative offices in Pune and Mumbai it has made enormous contributions in terms of public health policymaking process. CEHAT has come up with a number of alternative suggestions for National Health Policy 2001 and this has helped in assessing some very important issues related to primary health care, women and child health. The pertinent points of the document are stated below. CEHAT listed out some of the positive features of the NHP 2001 as:

- Direct, indirect acknowledgement of: High levels of morbidity and mortality; Poor functioning of Public Health Services; Gross under-funding of the Health Services.

- Takes note of higher public health expenditure in other countries; and its impact in health-status.
- Recommendation for doubling of central govt. health expenditure by 2010.
- Increased proportion of expenditure on primary health care. (55:35:10 formula)
- Envisages regulation of private sector and improvements in medical education.

Some of the Negative Features – General – Have Also been Listed

- No mention of Alma Ata Declaration and Primary Health Care Approach.
- No inter-sectoral linkages seen in determination of health-status and provision of health care services. Primary role of water, food, sanitation, environment etc. has been mentioned in the passing, at the end.
- Linkage between distorted development and morbidity pattern not recognized. No mention of double burden of old and new diseases; epidemiological polarization. Hence no policy to affect determinants of health through an inter-sectoral approach.
- No mention of special vulnerability of women due to the triple burden (pregnancy, child care, labour in unorganized sector) and the role of patriarchy.

Some of the Negative Features – Specific – Have been Listed As

- In Box 1, the achievements have not been compared with the goals for the year 2000, as envisaged in the 1983 policy.
- No indicator of malnourishment has been even mentioned. No mention of continued high prevalence of under-nourishment in children, anaemia in women.
- No critical analysis of overwhelming domination of F.P. program.
- No mention of the Community Health Worker for First Contact Care. No departure from doctor-centered model of medical care.

- No cognizance of opposition by women's and health-groups to injectable contraceptives. No change in the current unethical policy on this issue.
- Nothing on gender sensitization of health-care personnel and on health impact of domestic violence.
- Goals set in Box IV look arbitrary. They are unrealistic in the context of the experience so far.

Comprehensive Rural Health Project, (CRHP), established in Jamkhed Block of Ahmadnagar district and *Foundation for Research in Community Health, (FRCH)* established in Pune district of Maharashtra, have been initiated by stalwarts like Dr. Rajnikant Arole and Dr. N. H. Antia respectively, and for years have contributed in terms of a number of alternatives, suggestions, recommendations, through the research and community health work undertaken. These organizations have helped in formulation of new strategies for health communication, and health education in the field of reproductive health. Supporting the concept of barefoot doctors, i.e. training the local village health workers in providing with basic health care to the women has proved successfully in the long run.

Various Studies Undertaken By Researchers and Institutions Have Led to Several Suggestions and Recommendations for the Policy Making Process. Some of the Following Studies Have been Quoted Here:

1. Health Watch Trust in its study *"Community needs-based Reproductive and Child Health in India: Progress and Constraints"*, undertaken in 1998 in 9 states of India concluded that much of the lack of progress in the RCH program can be attributed to the inability of the program to bring about a shift in the attitudes of officials, service providers and communities. The training, along with the entire health system hierarchy, places no emphasis on anything other than quantitative achievements.[2]
2. Kulkarni S. and Parasuraman S. in a study *"Status of Maternal and Child Health in Maharashtra"*, presented in Workshop on Child Health and Family Planning Policy Issues in Maharashtra, 1997, reflected that the implementation of the program depends to a large extent on the performance of

Auxiliary Nurse Midwives(ANM), village health guides and Traditional Birth Attendants who as grassroots-level functionaries are the backbone of the MCH programme. It also examines the clients' reasons for not using ANC care; not feeling any need for ANC and not having the custom of seeking any ANC were reasons cited in both underdeveloped and developed states. Thus, persuading poor, illiterate, and older women seems to be a big challenge for field workers. The author recognizes the limitations of ANMs in terms of time and energy, and highlights the fact that the physical outreach of grassroots health workers is severely limited for lack of transport facilities. The study recommends and advocates IEC activities to convince these women of the need for ANC.[3]

3. Ramchandran V. and Visaria L. in their article *"Emerging issues in Reproductive Health"* published in *Economic and Political Weekly* in 1997 reflected that a range of recommendations was made specifically on ANMs, given the fact that they are the fulcrum around which all change revolves. If the ANM is to be the first and most accessible link between the people and the health system, she must be given the necessary tools, both medical and human, to sustain that position effectively. Capacity-building of male health workers was also recommended. The meetings also recommended involvement of women's groups in planning, implementing and monitoring the RCH program. It concluded that the relations between NGOs and GOs must be strengthened, especially in planning, implementing and monitoring RCH programs and the lack of information-sharing during the planning phases was lamented upon.[4]

4. Ravi Duggal in his paper on *"Health Sector Financing in Context of Women's Health"* presented at the National Seminar on Gender, Health and Reproduction, organised by ISST in Delhi 1995, expressed that in the last decade or so the health of women has been receiving special attention the world over. From the Nairobi UN Conference, through the ICPD at Cairo and to the recently concluded Beijing Conference, health and health care of women has been an important agenda item, which has taken a growing share of attention, and especially so Reproductive

Health. Beyond the above and some other occasional services like ante-natal care and abortion services (both within the context of Family Planning), very little else is available to women to address their general and other gender-specific health care needs. Of-course the informal sector practitioners do cater to some specific needs of women like abortions, white discharges, psychic problems (what patriarchal literature calls hysteria) etc., but very little of it is documented to enable a discussion or make comments. Women in India, and especially those in rural areas, given their general living conditions and the double burden on their shoulders, have never publicly voiced their concern over their reproductive, sexual and gynaecological health needs. Even something as obvious as menstruation is grossly neglected and this has serious consequences because many diseases in our country are related to blood loss and hence makes anaemia an extremely important concern of women's health which presently receives very little attention. The author concluded that in rural areas the PHC's and sub-centres are so poorly equipped for even these meagre services that the doctors and nurses are unwilling to risk even a normal delivery, ironically even tubectomy, the government's most favored 'health' program, is not available on demand to women at the PHC because it is done only in a camp where extra facilities/resources are made available. As regards spending specifically for women's' health care there is only the MCH program which gets merely 2% of the National Health budget, whereas, there is the Family Planning program which is targeted almost solely at women (tubectomies and IUD's) but it doesn't contribute much to women's' health care needs, if at all it has caused more harm than good.[5]

5. Kelley Lee, Louisiana Lush, Gill Walt and John Cleland London School of Hygiene and Tropical Medicine, University of London, Centre for Population Studies, DFID, Sexual and Reproductive Health Program in their study *"Family Planning policies and programs in eight low-income countries: A comparative policy"*, conclude regarding how policies are made, who makes them, and what policies are made, because much of the population policy literature has focused on the content of

policies-for example, what contraceptives to provide, which social groups to target, how to deliver Reproductive Health services and so on. These are clearly vital policy questions, however, there remains an important gap in the Population and Health Policy literature on the strategies that policy makers can use to introduce, develop and carry out new or changes in policy.[6]

6. Ravi Duggal in the paper presented at ICPD, Cairo, September 1994 *"Population and Family Planning Policy-a critique and a perspective"* reflected that the Official Population Policy and Program is based on the Malthusian belief that poverty in the third world countries is due to the large population of these countries. Each Five Year Plan in India has thus never failed to comment that India's development or growth has been the best possible with the given resources but uncontrolled population growth has acted as a retrogressive force. The IUD campaign did not shape up as anticipated and was more or less a failure, mainly because its prime concern was fulfilling targets and that the necessary medical and social backup support and follow-up was not available to women. In fact an Estimates Committee of the Lok Sabha (Parliament) was critical of the blind acceptance of foreign advice.[7]

7. Population Communications International and Ohio University in—*A Community Case Study of the Effects of a Radio Soap Opera on Gender Equality, Family Size, and Individual/ Collective Efficacy in India*, investigated the effects of a highly popular entertainment-education soap opera, *"Tinka Tinka Sukh"* (Happiness Lies in Small Things), designed to promote gender equality, Family Planning, and individual/collective efficacy, on a village community in India. It allowed the authors to understand the context of the radio program's reception, including the role of key opinion leaders in engendering strong audience effects.[8]

8. Population Communications International in a case study *"**Humraahi**": An Entertainment-Education Television Soap Opera to Promote Gender Equality in Marriage, Education, Socialization, and Family Life in India*, conducted a study of 4,000 people and in-depth interviews from 56 villages in North India, it

concluded that entertainment-education television soap operas can influence long-held attitudes about marriage and gender roles. These changes in audience members are stimulated by identification and para-social interaction with the characters, recognition of the consequences of the characters' behaviour, and interpersonal peer communication.[9]

9. A seminar held in India Habitat Centre, New Delhi in March 2003—*Global Agendas, Local Realities: Implications of Health Sector Reforms on Women's Access to Reproductive Health Services in India,* undertaken by Centre for Health and Gender Equity, reflected that concurrent to the ongoing process of health sector reforms, is the Reproductive Health agenda mandated by the International Conference on Population and Development (ICPD) in 1994. Part of the ICPD Program of Action can be seen as a reform of international health and population policies to ensure a focus on rights and equity issues within health, specifically Reproductive Health care, an area of specific neglect within primary health care service delivery. The ICPD mandate has placed Reproductive Health and rights on the map of Population Policy to ensure that population policies are linked to poverty reduction and improvements in individual well-being, especially the well-being and empowerment of women.

Political decentralization was examined as a process that has the potential to bring about substantial improvements in the health care delivery system as well as women's Reproductive Health care in Kerala. Conceptually, reform of the health care system was visualized as having three components in Kerala-Primary Health Care System, Panchayats and People's Planning Campaign and the community whose lives are most affected by and who have an active role to play in the reforms for their health care. It was found that Medical Officers' (MO) understanding of the Reproductive health (RH) approach was inadequate. The staff of the PHCs reported that there is less pressure to achieve Family Planning targets and more emphasis was on quality of care. The MOs felt that the RCH programme was in no way different from the earlier programmes. They provided several suggestions for improving women's access to health care including improving drug supplies, employing more female staff especially doctors and increasing availability of facilities to sterilize medical equipment. They recommended that private practice by government doctors should be regulated, duality of control over the staff by both the Directorate of Health Services and the PRIs needs to be addressed, and insurance mechanisms for poor patients need to be implemented. With respect to the RCH programme, two-third of the supervisors felt that it had made a difference, and 44% believed that it had the potential to involve more people compared to earlier programs. But all of them felt that it had increased their workload. The target free approach has not been adequately understood. The awareness of the community needs assessment, a hallmark of the Reproductive Health Approach, is inadequate even among those who had undergone RCH training. About one third of the workers and one-fifth of the supervisors did not know how to conduct a CNA.

The study observed that women hesitated to mention Reproductive Health problems to providers. Families are willing to invest available resources for acute reproductive health needs such as a difficult pregnancy or child birth but other reproductive health conditions such as white discharge, back pain, lower abdominal pain, joint paints, itching and menstrual irregularities are not taken seriously by either the women or their families. Even if they believe that contraceptives can adversely affect their health, the culturally prescribed gender role of taking responsibility for reproduction causes them to accept contraceptive responsibility. Some women believe that white discharge and other reproductive health problems like back ache and low abdominal pain are meant to be endured and cannot be cured.

10. Rao K.S. in the study *"Health care services in tribal areas of Andhra Pradesh: A public policy perspective"* reflected that the health of tribals is characterized by very high incidence of nutritional deficiency, maternal and under-5 mortality. There is a high prevalence of malaria and TB. These factors have serious consequences for the tribal population. The sex ratio is

declining at a faster rate and there is 75 per cent stunting/ wastage among tribal children. Centralized top-down planning and the inability of the tribals to articulate their need for health care services, are the two main reasons for an ambivalent public policy[10].

Various Studies Undertaken by Researchers and Institutions Have Led to Several Suggestions and Recommendations for the Policy Implementation Process. Some of the Following Studies Have been Quoted Here:

With regards to Communication Strategies applied in the field of Reproductive Health, the focus has been on Health Education (referred to as Information Education and Communication since ICPD 1994) programs. Reproductive Health education is operationally defined as scientifically correct information regarding anatomy of reproductive organs, fertility regulation methods, safe motherhood and child survival, consequences of teenage pregnancies, unsafe abortion and prevention of gynaecological disease, STD, HIV and AIDS etc which are conducive to Reproductive Health leading to human and social development.

1. M. K. Hassan, M. Jayaswal and P.Hassan, in their study *"Abstract Reproductive Health awareness in Rural Tribal – Female adolescents"* revealed that currently, a good deal of emphasis is being placed on women's Reproductive Health and now it is being increasingly realized that focus should be given on their awareness, individual needs, health and well being. The impetus for such emphasis was provided by the United Nations concern with the deplorable status of women as early as 1955, International Labour Organization (ILO) adopted a convention on Maternity Protection and subsequently the United Nations made a declaration in 1967 to ensure the universal recognition of the principles of equality between men and women. It organized the first World Women's Conference in 1975 in Mexico, which declared the decade of 1975-1985 as the decade for women. It created its voluntary fund in 1976 for promoting research on women, held second third and fourth World Conference on Women from 1980 to 1995 and published 'The World's Women-Trends and Statistics' in 1991 which was

a compilation of data on the condition of women throughout the world (UN, 1995).[11] Studies reported from other countries have indicated that women with Reproductive Health awareness begin child bearing later and end childbearing soon, give birth to few children, avoid unwanted pregnancies and adopt measures of control over their own physical, emotional and economic well being and also the well being of their off springs. On the other hand, lack of proper information or ignorance is the major factor of poor and miserable Reproductive Health.[12]

2. George A. and Nandraj S. in their study *"State of Health Care in Maharashtra – A Comparative Analysis"* concluded that Maharashtra has attained good health indicators, there is still a wide urban-rural as well as regional disparity. Public spending on health has decreased drastically since the First Five-year Plan, though the outlay for FP programmes has increased. The major part of the expenditure on health goes towards salaries and for the urban areas. Irrigation and power became top priority at the expense of health, probably because of the emergence of the powerful sugar lobby.

   The private sector has seen unregulated and unaccounted growth, which has in turn led to poor distribution, irrational and unethical practices and declining standards of care. NGOs have played an important role in health care in Maharashtra; they have experimented with innovative systems of health delivery, though only on a small scale, without any attempt at national or state-level impact. Though NGOs have better reach, they have been able to institute little change in people's participation in health. They have advocated user fees and have often weaned patients away from the government sector rather than from the private sector[13].

3. An empirical study – *District IEC Planning for RCH – Report 1 – by Institute of Health Management, Pachod, Aurangabad,* reflected that the rural audience was most comfortable with visuals, which were close to their reality and they identified themselves with it. Women stated a preference for interactive channels such as group meetings and home visits[14].

4. Khale M. and Dayalchand A. in their study *"Alternative approaches to MCH services"*, explained that in an attempt to evolve alternative approaches, IEC strategy was used for demand generation. The IHMP used women and children as agents of change to disseminate information in its program area. In these awareness camps they were given the opportunity for self-expression. Each camp ended with a decision and it was the responsibility of these women to implement the decision taken and to inform the community about it. This process helped generate demand and consequently created new norms in society. The health post also acted as a venue for group interaction and dissemination of information.[15]

5. Pachauri. S. in her study *"Relationship between AIDS and Family Planning programs: A rationale for developing integrated Reproductive Health services"*, reflected that although Reproductive Health is one of the primary concerns of Family Planning programs, problems related to sexuality and the sexual health needs of clients have not been explicitly addressed. RTIs have tended to remain invisible because of the 'culture of silence' that envelops them. The emergence of AIDS has brought about a renewed interest in STIs, which have been neglected in both developed and developing countries. Women's health advocates argue for comprehensive Reproductive Health services and contend that the present services must be redesigned as they do little to address the health needs of adolescents, the unmarried, the infertile, those with RTI and those with unintended pregnancies.[16]

6. Prakasamma M. in her study *"Implementing the RCH programme: Challenges before Nurses"* reflected that nursing education has been keeping up with changing trends in health policies and developments. The education and training of ANMs underwent hasty changes in order to meet the changing needs of these programs. ANMs were thus stripped off their midwifery competence over the course of time, although midwifery was the very reason for their emergence. The implementation of RCH policies now demand that these critical health care providers revert to their originally-designed set of skills and knowledge, and most important, change their

mindsets which have been geared towards 'target-oriented' Family Planning services for the last four decades. Their services are now expected to be more technically efficient, more concerned with quality, and gender-sensitive.[17]

7. Qadeer. I. in her study *"Reproductive Health: A Public Health Perspective"* reflected that the replacement of the concept of 'Women's Health' by 'Reproductive Health' by advocates of human development did not examine either the epidemiological basis of Reproductive Health or the reasons behind women's silence vis-à-vis reproductive health problems which would have revealed the immensity of the women's health problems and the social constraints on women's lives. Overlooking the causes of reproductive ill health, which lie outside conventional medical boundaries may lead to a superficial and medicalised intervention strategy and may thus fail to cure reproductive ill health. The life cycle approach, by identifying reproduction as the criterion for defining stages of life, actually medicalizes it and undermines the social processes at work. The compartmentalized perception of family and reproduction breaks the unity of production and reproduction in human societies. This then leads to isolated activism, which misses out on issues of socio-economic influence and the links between general health and Reproductive Health. It ignores the need to create simultaneous cushions in the social sphere while intervening at the family level.[18]

8. Pravesh Sharma (Special Senior Adviser, WFP and IFAD Facilitator in India) in his study *"IEC inputs for project implementation- Some lessons from Chattisgarh"*, reflected that IEC inputs are today widely recognised as a powerful and effective means of translating the sometimes arcane and complex messages of social interventions for the benefit of a diverse range of target groups. IEC become relevant and effective wherever the target group of the proposed intervention consists overwhelmingly of poor households, lives in a geographically dispersed area, is remote in terms of physical and other modern forms of communication and is poorly served by social services such as access to education, health, water and sanitation and, above all, information. Some modern communication theorists call this "social marketing", even

"social advertising". The use of modern technology (such as video, sound equipment etc.) should be restricted to the minimum and, wherever deployed, deployed in support of traditional forms of communication. Repeated doses of the intervention, with modifications based on feedback, are necessary to sustain the flow of communication between the project managers and the community.[19]

9. Ravi Duggal in his study *"India's Family Welfare Program in the Context of a Reproductive and Child Health Approach-A Critique and a Viewpoint"*, concluded that during the last decade or so the women's movements the world over, and especially in the west, have brought to center-stage women's Reproductive Health concerns, the origins possibly being the abortion debate in the United States of America. add to this the threat from Acquired Immuno Deficiency Syndrome (AIDS) and the population control lobby's supposed population bomb ticking away in third world countries leading to a new health policy prescription for countries who are seemingly endangering the world with their high fertility. India is one such country whose health policy is being reshaped in this new global context. At the outset it must be stated that 'Family Welfare' as a title is highly misleading because the entire effort of the concerned department is family planning, and that too mostly tubectomies. Other concerns of this department like child immunization, ante-natal care, abortions, deliveries, post-natal care etc. are only marginal. While in the fifties, the state did put in efforts at building an infrastructure to deliver basic health care, these were abandoned sometime in the sixties when population control started to become the cornerstone of India's health policy. The first casualty of this new approach was the Maternal and Child Health program with which the Family Planning program was integrated on the advise of a United Nations Advisory Mission to accommodate the loop program (the first ever IUCD program). The MCH program had at that time just taken off in the rural areas with the setting up of sub-centres and a large scale appointment of ANMs but both were hijacked by the newly created family planning department. From then on there was no looking back and population control kept getting an ever-increasing share of attention of health policy,

planning and resource allocations. The fate of all subsequent programs, like the Minimum Needs Program and integration of health workers under the multipurpose worker scheme, the Child Survival and Safe Motherhood program, the Community Health Volunteer Scheme, Universal Immunization Program etc. was the same-all ended up serving more the interests of the population control program than adhering to its own objectives. And it is this that makes up the misery and tragedy of health care, and specifically women's' health, in India. While recognizing the importance of Reproductive Health, especially in a country like India which still has relatively high fertility, an overwhelming proportion of deliveries being conducted at home, often under unhygienic conditions, a supposed unconcern for gynaecological morbidities, an embarrassingly high proportion of abortions being done outside the legal framework, etc. it becomes even more important to emphasize the need for making available comprehensive health services to all, and especially to women as a group for their special needs. And as mentioned earlier the danger of beginning with reproductive health(as a separate or special program) is narrowing down the focus to the uterus, precisely what the women's health movement wants to avoid.[20]

10. An evaluation of Danish Bilateral Assistance to health 1988-1997 in its chapter on – "Poverty and Cross Cutting Issues" reflected that the strategy of advocating community participation and including women as members of health committees has been attempted In India with varying degrees of success and that it has lead to tremendous success in Tamil Nadu community mobilization program on female infanticide.[21]

11. Shanti Conly in her study *"The missing billions"* reflected that in the final analysis the main responsibility for funding population programs falls squarely on the developing countries themselves. Indeed, about 75 per cent of costs are currently borne by them-primarily by governments, and to a lesser extent by private consumers. Since the Cairo conference, a number of governments, for example in India, Pakistan and Peru, appear to be increasing their funding in this area.[22]

12. *A World Bank Study* of initiatives for increasing community involvement in Karnataka and Tamil Nadu, reflected a detailed review of responsibilities of local governing bodies such as the Gram Panchayats and Zilla Parishads in initiating and implementing health programs. The recommendations highlight the need for including health as an area of priority, gender-sensitizing panchayat members on health issues and involving women in implementing health programs. The study also suggests proper dissemination of IEC (Information, Education and Communication) material to reach a wider audience so as to eradicate myths and misconceptions regarding health and reproductive matters apart from building up an information base.[23]

13. Avni Amin and Margaret E. Bentley in their study *"The Influence of Gender on Rural Women's Illness Experiences and Health-seeking Strategies for Gynaecological Symptoms"* concluded that community-based research on RTIs has shown that many women in India suffer a significant burden of morbidity from gynaecological symptoms and that gender inequalities, manifested through fertility, marriage and work norms, violence in marital relationships and poor psychological health, have resulted in rural Indian women accepting high thresholds of suffering, and not seeking treatment for their symptoms. The study recommended that RTI prevention and treatment efforts should be a part of a larger process of empowering women and men in which there is a discussion about reproductive, sexual and health rights[24].

14. *A Chikhaldara based non-governmental organisation (NGO)-Peoples Rural Education Movement (PREM)* in its survey found that lack of proper health care both by their families and the PHCs, has resulted in increasing number of tribal women giving birth to malnourished children. Inadequate basic health care, lack of elementary education and intensive land alienation of the indigenous people, improper childrearing practices, poor diet intake by the pregnant women, early marriages, poor spacing of children, lack of health education and awareness, lack of adequate income and purchasing power have were the main reasons for the precarious state of Maternal and Child Health in Melghat.

15. Bansal R. in his study *"Interns as health educators"* found that interns derived immense satisfaction from the experience of being trainers. Also based on the feedback of 25 mothers, the study inferred that the program had made some impact on the knowledge and attitudes amongst mothers who had consequently initiated actions[25].

16. Jejeebhoy S.J. in the study *"Addressing women's Reproductive Health needs: Priorities for the Family Welfare Program"* concluded that there is a need to decide strategies for making the Family Welfare program more woman-centered and holistic. The author takes stock of the prevalence of maternal mortality and its causes. The extent of reproductive morbidity is noted. Maternal health activities are unbalanced, focusing on immunization and the provision of iron and folic acid, rather than on sustained care of women or on the detection and referral of high-risk cases.

    The risk elements affecting Reproductive Health like malnutrition attributable to gender disparities; vulnerability and neglect of adolescent girls; contraceptive patterns and overemphasis on terminal methods and female methods; poor quality of health care services; poorly-addressed health information needs and sex education needs, specially of women and adolescents have been identified[26].

17. Jejeebhoy S.J. in the study *"Adolescent sexual and reproductive behaviour"* concluded that there are an estimated 190 million 10-19-year-old adolescents in India, over one-fifth of the population. Adolescent marriage and adolescent fertility are disturbingly high. Unlike other countries, adolescent fertility in India occurs mainly within the context of marriage. Half of all women aged 15-19 have experienced a pregnancy or a birth. Apart from early marriage and fertility, there is little information on other aspects of adolescent reproductive health problems. Adolescent sexual behaviour, sexual awareness and attitudes remain poorly-explored topics. Both unmarried and married women are vulnerable to being unprotected from pregnancy and sexually transmitted infection[27].

REFERENCES

1. *Suggestions for National Health Policy 2001*, (Mumabi, CEHAT, 2001).

2. Health Watch Trust, Community Needs-based Reproductive and Child Health in India: Progress and constraints, (New Delhi, 1999).

3. Kulkarni S. and Parasuraman S., '*Status of Maternal and Child Health in Maharashtra*', Paper presented in Workshop on Child Health and Family Planning Policy Issues in Maharashtra, 1997.

4. Ramachandran V. and Visaria L. 'Emerging Issues in Reproductive Health', *Economic and Political Weekly, 1997*.

5. Ravi Duggal, *Health Sector Financing in Context of Womens' Health*, (New Delhi, ISST, 1995.

6. Kelley Lee, Louisiana Lush, Gill Walt and John Cleland, *Family Planning Policies and Programs in Eight Low-income Countries: A Comparative Policy*, London School of Hygiene and Tropical Medicine, University of London, 2000.

7. Ravi Duggal, *'Population and Family Planning Policy: A Critique and a Perspective'* Paper Presented at International Conference on Population and Development, Cairo, September 1994. (Mumbai – CEHAT – 1994).

8. Population Communications International and Ohio University, *'A Community Case* Study of the Effects of a Radio Soap Opera on Gender Equality, Family Size, and Individual/Collective Efficacy in India,' Ohio University, USA, 2002.

9. Population Communications International, *'Humraahi': An Entertainment-Education Television Soap Opera to Promote Gender Equality in Marriage, Education, Socialization, and Family Life in India*, New York, 2002.

10. Rao K.S. Health Care Services in Tribal Areas of Andhra Pradesh: A Public Policy Perspective *Economic and Political Weekly*, 1998.

11. M.K.Hassan, M. Jayaswal and P.Hassan, 'Abstract Reproductive Health Awareness in Rural Tribal Female Adolescents" Research Study, Ranchi University, 2001.

12. M.K.Hassan et.al., n 11.

13. George A. and Nandraj S. "State of Health Care in Maharashtra—A Comparative Analysis", *Economic and Political Weekly*, 1993.

14. Institute of Health Management, *District IEC Planning for RCH, Report 1*, Aurangabad, Maharashtra, 1998.

15. Khale M. and Dayalchand A., Alternative Approaches to MCH Services, *Indian Paediatrics*, Aurangabad, Maharashtra, 1991.

16. Pachauri S., "Relationship Between AIDS and Family Planning Programmes: A Rationale for Developing Integrated Reproductive Health Services", *Health Transition Review*, 1994.

17. Prakasamma M, "Implementing the RCH Program: Challenges Before Nurses", *Indian Journal of Nursing & Midwifery*, 1998.

18. Qadeer I., "Reproductive Health: A Public Health Perspective", *Economic and Political Weekly*, 1998.

19. Pravesh Sharma, "IEC inputs for Project implementation- Some Lessons from Chattisgarh", *WFP – IFAD*, India, 2002.

20. Ravi Duggal, "India's family Welfare Program in the Context of a Reproductive and Child Health Approach-A Critique and a Viewpoint', *MFC Bulletin, No. 234-235*, Mumbai, Sept-Oct 1996.

21. Danida, Evaluation of Danish Bilateral Assistance to Health 1988 - 1997, Poverty and Crosscutting issues, (New Delhi, 1998).

22. Shanti Conly, 'The Missing Billions', *People and the Planet* –, Vol. 6 No. 1.

23. World Bank/ CINI (Child in Need Institute), *Study of Initiatives for Increasing Community Involvement in Karnataka and Tamil Nadu*, New Delhi, 1998.

24. Avni Amin and Margaret E. Bentley in Their Study *"The Influence of Gender on Rural Women's Illness Experiences and Health-seeking Strategies for Gynaecological Symptoms"* New Delhi, Visiaar Publications 1996.

25 Bansal R. in his Study *'Interns As Health Educators'* World Health Forum, 1995.

26. Jejeebhoy S.J. in the Study 'Addressing Women's Reproductive Health Needs: Priorities for the Family Welfare Program' *Economic and Political Weekly*, 1997.

27. Shireen Jejeebhoy, *Women's Education, Autonomy, and Reproductive Behaviour: Experience form Developing Countries*, Oxford, Clarendon press 1995.

7

Public Health Care Programs in Maharashtra

Introduction

In the present chapter the analysis of the impact is done at two levels.

(a) Assessment of program implementation done by the Maharashtra state government.

(b) Analysis of the several public reports, news paper reports and personal interviews.

Level I: Program Implementation by the State Government

Policy Highlights and its Analysis: The Maharashtra State Population Policy 2000 states the following as major concerns: Low average age at marriage for girls resulting in higher teenaged fertility; low acceptance of spacing methods; and very high prevalence of "Son Preference". Along with this it also declares the strategic themes like Convergence of Service Delivery at village levels; empowering women for improved health and nutrition; increased participation of men in Planned Parenthood; research in RCH; and Information, Education and Communication. The IEC strategy stated in the State Population Policy with regards to the reproductive health aspects focuses on age at marriage; medical termination of pregnancy; importance of safe delivery practices for safe motherhood; value of a girl child and who determines the sex of a child; and adolescent health. Though the policy states all the appropriate concerns and appropriate measures, what is needed more is the appropriate mechanisms for implementation of the same.

The several mechanisms for monitoring and successful implementation of the policy like: State Population Commission, Coordination Committee and State Population Women Commission at the State level; Divisional Population Coordination Committee at the divisional level; and Population Coordination Committee and Population Monitoring Committee at the district level; have been presented. However, it fails to notify the actual grassroots level mechanisms and the models for strict inspections. The analysis of these mechanisms and the lacunae in the same are stated in the sections related to functioning of IEC unit at district level instituted in the District Health Office.

Panchayati Raj and Constitutional amendments: As per the 73rd and 74th amendments to the Constitution, the Panchayati Raj institutions are seen as an important means of furthering decentralized planning and program implementation. The Panchayati Raj system of Maharashtra state also ensures the complete executive powers for overall development to the Chief Executive Officer of the district. One of the principal features of the Panchayati Raj in Maharashtra has been the separation of the executive function from the deliberative function. The policy making function has been entrusted to the elected representatives of the people. One third of the elected seats at all the three levels of the Panchayati Raj are reserved for women who can give a push to the health of women and children. Accordingly, a number of IEC and awareness programs have been undertaken by the Panchayati Raj Institutions especially with reference to the superstitions in the Korku philosophy and efforts are ongoing to change this superstitious mindset. There has been a shortage of resource material and methods as well as some very crucial aspects like lack of knowledge and understanding of Korku language. However, it was pointed out[1] that today efforts are being made to educate the concerned officials in their language with the aim to reach them as a better strategy in the long run.

Findings of National Family Health Survey-II- 1998-99: The NFHS II reflected various findings directly connected to the Reproductive

Health of women. It revealed that knowledge of the pill, IUD and condom has improved, but use of these methods (only 8% of users) still remains low, these are useful for women who want to space their next birth, a preference expressed by 10 per cent of women; exposure to media is moderately high, about 62% saw or heard a message on family planning during the months before the survey, nevertheless, about 2 out of 5 women are not regularly exposed to family planning messages; among women currently using contraception, few were told about other methods or side effects of their current method, this reflects a low quality of services; many women are still not involved in personal health care decisions, only half of women report having a voice in decision about their own health; women's nutritional status is poor, about two –fifths of women are malnourished and nearly one third of pregnant women have moderate to severe Anemia, compared to non pregnant women.

The above mentioned findings of the survey provide with a clear guideline for the policy makers as well as implementers, and hence necessary efforts have been designed by the state Health Department, however, more emphasis still has to be paid on the women's role in decision-making with regards to her health.

Focus required on Reproductive Health Problems: The implementation of various programs by the state government with the help of IEC techniques, information material, personal meetings and counseling, has helped in achieving success of 52% of women's involvement in following various Family Planning methods, reduction of birth rate to 21.1 per thousand, increase in the couple protection rate, spacing between two children and reduction in the age of marriage. Though this is an excellent performance in the field of Family Welfare by the state, the responsibility of tackling and providing resources to solve reproductive health problems is also entirely with the Family Welfare wing of the Directorate of Health Services, as there is no separate wing for Reproductive Health.

The crucial aspects like RTI/STI and reproductive disorders are being handled by the projects implemented by the Maharashtra State AIDS Control Society (MSACS). This is done with the syndromic approach taken by the MSACS, wherein the Doctors and ANMs are trained. With all these measures undertaken for RTI /STI, however, still more established mechanisms are required because knowledge, symptoms and expression of the same by the women is more important. Therefore, the need is to train the health workers in identifying the problems of women and talking with them with utmost confidence and clarity.

RCH Camps – A camp based approach still continues. In order to have an easy access for the treatment of RTI/STI, Disease Diagnostic Camps are conducted under the scheme. The following type of services are provided in the camp: Information counseling and services; Contraceptive methods; Menstrual regulation; MTP services; Gynecological problems (RTI/STI); and Adolescent problems. The idea behind these camps is to cater to the women who lack the availability of services by gynecologists at the village level, as there is a dearth of these services in remote rural areas. However, at the same time it should also be noted that diagnostic camps are still looked at by people as the target based camps undertaken for tubectomies/laparoscopies and vasectomies; camps do not cater to the emergency issues; the non availability of some needy women during the period of camp definitely acts as their loss; most important, the women are not as open and frank in the camp atmosphere as they would be in a regular clinic atmosphere; and sometimes the women avoid such camps due to the taboo attached to such camps. It is extremely important to note that despite a number of services arranged by the Public Health Department, the services of the gynecologists should also be considered as one of the most crucial services and appropriate and regular availability for the same seems to be a must in case the major reproductive health problems of the women are to be catered for.

Financial Provisions – In the post ICPD scenario, new programs have been initiated with the financial assistance of various funding organizations like WHO, World Bank, UNICEF, European Union and GTZ. This is just not limited to the program implementation but has also catered to the infrastructural development. The problem anticipated is one of sustainability, as future assistance on a regular basis cannot be completely assured from any agency, nor is there any non-plan allocation made by the central government. Health being a state subject, its sustainability is dependant on allocations made by the state. Unless these programs are a part of the plan budget the states find it difficult to sustain it. Further, states have a tendency to divert program funds away from components they are earmarked for and this is largely due to the restricted role that states play in policy-making and planning.

Implementation of Area Projects: Some of the area projects implemented in several districts like the RCH – Sub – Project – RTI/STI, District Nasik; Area project in RCH – Wardha; Integrated Population and Development Project(UNFPA) in Thane, Dhule, Nandurbar, Chandrapur, Gadchiroli, Wardha and the Corporations, Thane, Pune, Kalyan, Ulhasnagar and Bhiwandi; are being implemented effectively as pilot projects, however, with their completion of first phases it is important that these pilot projects need to be replicated in other districts. If the duplication or extension of the financial assistance is not possible, at-least the models and strategies of implementation need to be replicated.

Merging of Earlier Programs with the RCH Program and its Output: Though the Maternal and Child Health program as well as Child Survival and Safe Motherhood Program has been merged with the existing RCH program in the state, a number of officials still maintain an opinion that the new RCH program is no different from the earlier ones and that it only has a new name. One of the officials pointed out that there is a need to change the strategies and mechanisms of the program implementation rather than having new names. At the same time a lot of sensitization of the government officials is required in order to bring in changes in attitudes and practices[2].

Infrastructural Development and its Utilization: The state has developed a large health infrastructure in the form of physical facilities, staff and equipment. Every district has a required number of Rural Hospitals, PHCs and Sub-centers. However, while visiting these infrastructural sites, one notices that they stand there as silent structures, because very little utilization of these structures is extended to the general public as they remain closed most of the times. It is difficult to judge whether the change in this situation can come from sensitization or penalization of the officials concerned. But it is necessary for the government to adopt both the methods and ensure the required service delivery from these infrastructures.

Family Welfare Program of Government of Maharashtra: Despite the adoption of the target based approach since the year 1996, the performance of the Family Welfare program is still measured in terms of the sterilization conducted. While the performance is mainly through female sterilization operations, the Population Policy is now giving stress on male sterilizations, therefore, a special scheme promoting No Scalpel Vasectomy (NSV) is being implemented.

Implementation of Pre Natal Diagnostics Techniques (Regulation and Prevention of Misuse)(PNDT) Act: This Act came in to force on 1st January 1996. The falling sex ratio in the state from 934 in the 1991 census to 922 has compelled the state to take stringent measures against the genetic counseling centers and doctors violating the act. The state has accordingly raided a number of clinics and filed cases against the culprits, the two most famous cases are one that occurred in Satara district and the Malpani case in Mumbai. The raids have definitely deterred the practicing doctors from undertaking the illegal activities.

Implementation of Special Schemes of Melghat Pattern: The schemes like Matrutwa Anudan Yojana, Flying squads for the inspection of work, Dai Training, Pada Swayamsevak Scheme, Deputation of Pediatricians during the epidemic prone period, Appointment of Honorary Doctors, Establishment of Paediatric Intensive Care Unit, and Use of Thermo-Cole Boxes are some of the most appropriate and need based schemes for the area. It is important to note that the government has also ensured the changes in the strategy of implementation and flexibility with regards to the schemes based on their performance indicators, for example, in case of Matrutwa Anudan Yojana, which initially started with provision of Rs. 800 as cash amount was later changed to a break-up of food-grains and medicines worth Rs. 400 each, due to the reports that the money was not being utilized for buying.

IEC Material produced in the state: A brochure of IEC Bureau displays a list of material prepared by the IEC Bureau in last three years. It would be seen that 198 items are produced with 12, 043, 283 number of copies. What needs to be enquired is whether, the amount of material prepared by the State IEC Bureau is enough and covers/ caters to all the issues related to Public Health in the state.

IEC programs undertaken in Amrawati district: Table 5.11 of Chapter Five provides an overview of IEC activities in Amrawati district. It would be seen from the data presented in the table that totally 325 film shows have been undertaken in last two years, whereas, 200 shows were proposed to be completed in 2002-2003. It also shows that totally 15,000 display publicity were undertaken in last two years, whereas 10,000 display publicity were proposed in the year 2002-2003. Further it shows, that totally 297 exhibitions were conducted in last two years, whereas, 260 exhibitions were proposed to be undertaken in the year 2002-2003.

Level II: Analysis of the Public Reports, News Paper Reports and Personal Interviews

A number of secondary data as well as newspaper reports have been explored. A number of government officials involved in the policy making and policy implementation process have been interviewed. Apart from this the entire functioning process of the State IEC Bureau at the head quarters level and the functioning of IEC units at the district level has been studied.

Policy Making: The policy making process generally comprises of involvement of the Director General and other technical experts from the Directorate of Health Services, who prepare the draft, due to their technical knowledge, and further the discussion is held with the Ministry to finalize the same. The role of the Directorate of Health Services is in technically guiding and providing inputs to the policy makers and further implementation has to be looked into entirely by the DHS. The officials at (DHS) are generally involved in preparing various proposals to be sent to the state government for decision-making. The Director General, Health Services, argued that it was extremely necessary to develop a Public Health approach while everybody is involved in the day- to-day work.[3]

There are special action plans designed for have for the 5 ITDP districts – Thane, Nasik, Nadurbar, Amravati and Gadchiroli. Since these special action plans have been successful, the pattern of schemes implemented in these areas is further being replicated in the other 10 tribal districts. The health policies made for and implemented in Amravati district are important because after 1993, the number of policies and schemes were implemented came to be known as "Melghat Pattern". This looked as a complete package of schemes to be implemented and replicated in another tribal district of the state.

Policy Implementation Process: The DGHS opined that the policy implementation process was smooth enough but that was mainly due to pressure put on all the implementers. The present focus is on inter-sectoral coordination and collaboration. The coordination between ICDS, Food and Drugs department, Civil Construction, EGS, Road and Infrastructure Development, Women and Child Welfare Department and many more departments is continuously sought for. This was one of the main strategies applied in Amravati district after the infant mortality crisis.

The State Minister for Health opined that upgrading of infrastructural and technical services in few hospitals has been the latest implementation plan in the state.

Adequacy of Policies: Most of the officials opined that the policies made by both the Center and the States are adequate enough and are suitable for the purpose and goals. One would have to look at the results provided by these policies. The proof that the policies have worked and helped us attain the goals like the reduction in decadal growth of the state (in 1981-91 it was 25.73%, this reduced to 22.57% in 1991-2001) explains the adequacy of the policies made. Other such examples like improvement in literacy rates, reduction in IMR have ensured that policies framed and measures taken are definitely fetching results opined Principal Secretary, Family Welfare[44] Interview of Dr. Manmohan Singh, Principal Secretary, Family Welfare, Public Health Department, Maharashtra State.

Adequacy of Schemes: Most of the schemes are framed and initiated by the government of India and some are developed from the state's perspective. The schemes designed are very useful and really beneficial to people, however the major problem is the generation of resources, as well as sustainability of these schemes. Again the success of most of these schemes is due to a lot of pressure as the efforts undertaken in the entire process of implementation of the scheme and the resources generated[5].

Importance of Region Specific Policies: Applicability of policies is commonly done in all the regions. What differs is the approach in each region and accordingly the activities also differ. The state machinery definitely possesses a lot of flexibility in doing so, the classic example is that of evolution of Melghat pattern over a period of time, that considering the prevailing conditions, the policies were accordingly designed, set and implemented opined the DGHS, Maharashtra.

Suggestions for Structuring of New Policies: The DGHS talked about the requirement of more clarity in setting new goals, as these set goals have to be at the same time compared and matched with the existing achievements and policies. There is a need to set clear indicators and these need to be defined for each activity to be implemented[6]. Along with the structuring of new policies, the most important aspect to be considered is the sufficiency of resources to implement the same, as in a large number of policies, this aspect is overlooked by the central government and when it comes to implementation by the state government, due to lack of resources, the policies do not yield results. Apart from this, the discontinuation of grants from the Central Government to the Post Partum Centers, recently has resulted into a financial loss of Rs. 66 Crores to the State Government[7].

Further, in structuring of new policies for health, everything has to be coordinated with education, as without the extension of education in our country, it is really difficult to achieve results[8].

Suggestions for Better Implementation: To a large extent the central government has failed to understand the problems and issues of the peripheral and grass roots workers, at the same time we find that it is equally challenging to explain the policy implementation process to the peripheral and middle level authorities, there is a need to increase the connectivity between the top level, middle level and grass-root level officials in order to help enable a smooth implementation process opined the DGHS[9].

Some of the officials[10] talked of the difficulties that occur in the implementation process. Firstly, a lot of bureaucratic delays occur in the renewal of schemes each year. Any scheme designed, should be let for implementation for at least forthcoming five years, however the uncertainty of political commitment to most of the schemes, meant that they have to be renewed every year. The delay in renewal obviously leads to delay in actual implementation at the grass-root level. Secondly, lack of inter-departmental coordination especially at the grass root level causes a lot of problems. Thirdly, in the remote tribal areas, there are very few NGOs, that cooperate with the government, in-fact most of the time, these are involved in investigating and cross-checking the governmental efforts and creating more obstacles in the implementation process, the NGOs fail to understand that their job is uni-purpose whereas the PHC has to provide with multipurpose services. It is also important to note that the workload for the grass-root level workers is quite heavy; if one studies the actual work of each staff, one finds that everybody is having a supervisory role and the only person to work and supervised is the ANM. It is extremely pathetic to talk about the village level situation, here the field level staff of health workers, health assistants, LHVs, ANMs, and the anganwadi staff is supposed to work together, but one rarely gets to see this collaboration. Once the pregnant and lactating mothers along with their children are there in Anganwadi, every service including the day to day health education can be extended here. Instead of applying this technique for reaching out to the potential audience, the reasons like lack of time and inability to cater to such a large number of women at one time are given.

Officials also talked about the realities of the Public Health Department, which need to be brought in front of the common man. For example the Medical Officer (MO) at PHC despite drawing a handsome salary and all the other facilities as per the Fifth Pay Commission, the MO is disinterested in practicing for few hours every day and catering to an OPD of maximum 30 village families at one time. So naturally, if the people do not receive day-to-day services, they can never expect any service in an emergency. It is also pathetic to find that most of the staff from the PHC, be it Health Assistant or MPW, manage to give injections and medicines at local level and draw an extra income from the villagers[11].

There exist a number of difficulties in the implementation of IEC programs, due to lack of experts and manpower for the same. The Pada Worker scheme should be extended as it is easier to assign the work to locally available persons and train them for the required tasks. Most of the procedures are time consuming; these should be relaxed and will automatically lead to solutions for problems in implementation. The government has to seriously adopt new strategies with regards to the non-availability of staff and experts, because otherwise the quality of care suffers. The emphasis should be on developing inter-personal skills, maintenance of registers, record keeping, provision of vehicles and communication facilities.

The most recent strategy implemented is to replace males by female workers as experience has shown that efficiency is more assured in case of female workers.

Suggestion for Communication Strategies in Reproductive Health: Various documents and drafts have been prepared, meetings have been undertaken, a lot of training is imparted to the concerned staff and officials, however it is felt that the concept of IEC, is inappropriately understood by the implementers. IEC can be called a success only when it becomes a part of people's life rather than just an episode that they have watched and listened to. Hence, this is a process and behaviour change is very necessary. The community acceptance needs to be systematized[12]. The Principal Secretary Family Welfare expressed "We cannot and should not deny sex education to our adolescents, sufficient RCH and Family Life Education as a curriculum should be regularly imparted to the students, the end purpose will be achieved, literature and resources are already available and this only needs to be incorporated, religion and other factors should not be brought into the picture, IEC is equally important for the opinion moulders. In our country even the politicians are feeling shy, states like Andhra Pradesh and Tamil Nadu have taken the lead and have been successful in their IEC campaigns and the government has not collapsed, implementation has to be percolated from top to bottom"[13].

In Melghat the local folk media has played a good role, further the importance of right age of marriage, limited pregnancies and spacing of births is being undertaken through the IEC activities. Participatory measures are required everywhere, also in policy making, the onus is on people too, government can only create infrastructures, the initiative to utilize the services and ensuring its proper work, has to come from people, explained the Principal Secretary Public Health.

The State Minister for Health, did give an opinion that despite all the efforts in preparation and distribution of IEC material, the dissemination of this material is not up to the mark and there needs to be more training and sensitization of the field level workers regarding dissemination of information, the seriousness and the need of the day has to be conveyed. Apart from this he also opined that the inspection machinery to check these measures is not very effective and this also has to be considered soon, though the inspections take place randomly, the negligence and carelessness continues to exist[14].

Comprehensive Health Policy: The Maharashtra State Policy on Reproductive Health has been covered in the policy documents on Family Welfare and Population Policy, which are in line with the National Policies. With regards to RCH, the two documents, Government of India Manual on Community Needs Assessment Approach in Family Welfare Program and a manual on Reproductive and Child Health Program. The state has not yet produced a comprehensive policy document covering all the aspects of Public Health including Reproductive Health, Dr. Subhash Salunke, the Director General of Health Services, Maharashtra agreed that there was a need to frame a comprehensive Public Health policy and the need to go project by project in this document. He argued that the State possesses experience and knowledge to do so but at the same time it lack time and people with analytical inclination and skills and hence no attempt had been made in drafting this document.

Pre Natal Diagnostics Techniques (Regulation and Prevention of Misuse Act) 1994: The female ratio in Maharashtra State has come down to 922 in the 2001 census as compared to 934 in the 1991 census. The Supreme Court has already directed all the States to take stringent measures against the mis-utilization of the PNDT act. After a thorough analysis of the IEC material prepared by the Maharashtra State IEC Bureau, it is appreciable to note that a lot of material is geared towards the task of creating awareness and educating parents and concerned people regarding the issues covered in the act and the ill effects as well as penalties incurred in case of misuse.

People's Belief in TBA Continues: Normally, the PHCs are well equipped with the for conducting institutional deliveries, however, people in the rural and tribal areas still have trust in the Dais or the Traditional Birth Attendants, and hence prefer to go in for a home/ non institutional delivery. Part of this preference may be a product of the non-availability of Doctors in the PHCs. In the Chikhali village of Chikhaldara block, one of the dais and the women being catered by her expressed regarding the expertise the traditional dais possess with regards to difficult deliveries and talked about a recent episode in their village, wherein an ANM was assisted by the same dai in a home delivery as the baby had expired in the womb and due to emergency at night, there was no transportation available to take ANM to the PHC and hence her case had to be handled by the dai. Presently, the Health Department has adopted the strategy of training the dais and also conducting meetings and workshops along with them, this has definitely helped but at the same time it is equally necessary that confidence-building measures are undertaken, so that the villagers approach the ANM and develop confidence in an institutional delivery.

People's Response to NSV Campaign: The government has launched a special program with the emphasis on the male sterilization called Non Scalpel Vasectomy; however this program has a good response and success rate in the urban areas and not in rural areas. Rigorous efforts are required to reduce the burden of sterilization from the shoulders of women in rural and tribal areas. Even while talking to the couples in reproductive age every few men really knew about the recently launched program of NSV.

Skill Based Training: Under the RCH program a lot of skill based training is extended to the health personnel, and it is appreciated that the technical training imparted has in lot many ways helped in improving the service delivery in the villages. However, at the same time it is necessary that along with the technical training, the sensitization to understand and counsel the women patients on several of their reproductive health problems is done. It is important to note here that talking to a woman about her health and creating confidence in her by knowing her day-to-day reproductive disorders is one of the best strategy to ensure the impact of IEC.

Lack of Clarity on Budget Spent for RCH Component: There appears to be no clarity on the budget being spent by the Central Government on the RCH component, as despite the financial assistance, a lot of funds are extended in kind in terms of material and medicines, and many times the valuation process does not even take place. It has also been studied that many times the material sent may or may not be useful on one hand or even may or may not be worth utilizing due to it having been expired or was culturally inappropriate material.

Distribution of IEC Material and Information Dissemination: The Maharashtra State IEC Bureau is located in Pune. The IEC bureau provides with entire IEC material and inputs for public health components in the total state. Most of the IEC material is based on the communicable diseases and the Pre Natal Diagnostics Techniques (Regulation and Prevention of Misuse) Act, mainly relating with equality for both the sexes, respect for the girl child, and ill effects of sex determination tests etc. A democratic and participatory procedure is adopted (as mentioned in Chapter Five) for material preparation. The distribution of material is also well managed, but there exists lacunae with regards to the dissemination of this information. The several reasons for these lacunae could be lack of inclination and understanding of the officials to disseminate the material at required places, disinterest and non importance accrued with this activity and lack of supervision and inspection by the concerned authorities placed in the IEC Bureau. One of the officials informed that at the time of inspection, the tin posters in one of the sub-centers were utilized for a rooftop rather than displayed for the people. It was also pointed out that the dissemination of information largely depends on the interest of the DHO and the DEMO in doing so; otherwise, the material lies around without being utilized[15].

Emphasis on Print Material for IEC: Due to lack of electricity and manpower in rural areas, the emphasis is on the print media and very little material is prepared in the form of electronic media. Most of the IEC material prepared is in print form. Here too, if the audience is literate then it is easier to understand, as many times the pictures on the posters are not enough to convey the message. This was observed in Melghat, wherein the literacy level is very low.

Importance of the Language in IEC: Most of the material is prepared in the state language, Marathi, with exceptional cases of Hindi language. The tribal areas and many border areas of Maharashtra demand that the IEC material be prepared in local language. With regards to Melghat the local language is Korku, which is more influenced by Hindi. Apart from few sayings in Korku language painted on the sanitary blocks or school building, most of the displayed material throughout the region is in Marathi Language. Exceptional efforts in developing folk dramas, street plays and songs in Korku language have been undertaken by Mr. Mhatne, the District Education and Media Officer of Amravati district; however this needs to be supported by the State IEC Bureau.

Lack of Monitoring with Regards to Mahila Swasthya Sanghs: An important component of the implementation of programs in reproductive health is the program of formulating Mahila Swasthya Sanghs, here the women are to formulate a group and have monthly meetings and discussions on various issues, the Anganwadi and the ANM is suppose to collaborate with these groups, and these groups can be used as direct platforms for a number of IEC activities. However, the scheme lacks inspection, monitoring and involvement from concerned officials[16].

Reduction in the Number of Health Bulletins: The State IEC Bureau produces a monthly health bulletin, which is circulated to most of the offices at the Zilla Parishad level. Over a period of time, there has been a reduction in the production and subsequently distribution of these bulletins from 65,000 to 35,000 copies every month, the reason being lack of financial resources. In normal case, the production should have increased as growing numbers of government officials and village level functionaries need to be circulated with this bulletin, but unfortunately, the decrease in the quantity has further resulted in deprivation of this bulletin to a lot of people who earlier benefited from it.

District IEC Unit and the Staff: Each district has its own IEC unit, stationed in the DHO office, lead by the District Education and Media Officer (DEMO), assisted by an Artist, Projectionist, Driver, Health Assistant, and a Peon. The recent status of staff available in IEC units of all the 33 districts in October 2003 reflects a very shocking picture of the personnel involved in the IEC. Out of all the posts in 33 districts, only 7 districts have the position of DEMO filled, in other districts the post remain vacant, there are totally 11 artists, 10 projectionists, and 21 drivers in all 33 districts with no Health assistants and Peons in any district. After looking at the said statistics, keeping very high expectations in the performance and impact of IEC activities is extremely ironical.

Need to Avoid Duplication of Efforts: Apart from the regular implementation of government programs, the special area projects supported by external/international funding agencies, the health programs implemented by NGOs and many programs are sometimes implemented in the same area with same objectives and similar focus. It is thus more practical to ensure collaboration of all these efforts at district level, so that duplication of efforts in some areas and at the same time absolute lack of efforts in some areas is avoided.

The Response of Korkus to Health Programs: Initially in 1993 a lot of difficulties were encountered by the Health Department in implementing some programs like, the compulsion by the state government to hospitalize the children affected from malnutrition In such cases at least one parent of the child had to be with the child, and since the parents were not accustomed to something like this they would run away from the hospital leaving the child behind. After some time, police were posted in the hospitals to ensure that the parents stayed back with their children, even then this was a very difficult task to implement. A few years ago the tribal people in this area could never accept the idea of immunization or even approaching the PHC for their ailments. But, over a period of time the women as well as children are taken for immunization, there is a faster registration of ANC cases and people also approach PHC normally even in emergencies. Apart from all this change, the special schemes in the area have helped the tribal in upgrading their health status.

Designing of New Strategies for Emergency Obstetric Care: The DHO, Amrawati spoke about the new strategy developed in Melghat with regards to emergency obstetric care. Since Chikhaldara and Dharni are 100 and 150 Kilometers away from the district head quarters respectively, there are no facilities available for a Caesarian section, whereas some facility for the same is available at Dharni. Since every type of delivery should be treated as emergency, a Calendar Method is being implemented, the cases of women in their last trimester along with the day, date and location are noted on the calendar which gives an immediate view about their requirements of ANCs and emergency care, this has helped a lot in tackling the difficult pregnancies as the PHC officials are on their watch regarding each case.

Supervision, Reporting and Inspection: Strengthening of supervision in Melghat became a necessity and emergency in the wake of infant mortality crisis in 1993. This was also demanded into the PIL filed by Sheela Barse in 1993. The efforts taken thereby to improve supervision, reporting and inspection reflect visible results today. Especially the appointment of a special Flying Squad to monitor and inspect the work of the health officials specifically in the Chikhaldara and Dharni blocks of Melghat has fetched results in terms of service delivery.

Leadership amongst Korkus: Amongst the tribal, a sense of leadership has emerged over a period of years, now one finds Korku leaders and people making their demands through their leaders. Nevertheless, the Korku leadership has not influenced the implementation of health programs. The Korkus discussed that many cases were traced from the villages regarding frauds and partiality, but the Korku leaders have not been able to do much about it.

Efforts of NGOs and Other Agencies: Melghat Mitra; Peoples Rural education Movement; Lok Arogya Margdarshan Pratishthan are some of the Melghat based NGOs working on issues related to tribal development. Melghat Mitra, is a group of individuals, which works exclusively for the betterment of the Korkus, in terms of preventive health care, environmental sanitation and nutrition to needy children. A Chikaldhara-based NGO, Peoples Rural Education Movement (PREM), in collaboration with government agencies, is actively engaged in protecting vulnerable children from disease and deaths in Melghat. Lok Arogya Margdarshan Pratishthan, works in the field of Reproductive Health, and has implemented the RCH project supported by the Government of India; the focus is mainly upon information sharing with the women regarding their basic and routine reproductive health problems. Though a number of NGOs have emerged in the post 1993 period, most of them exist on paper and one finds it difficult to trace them in the field, and the local people do not recognize these organizations.

The Difficult Triangle – "Forest-Livelihood-Health": For centuries together, the Korkus have been directly dependent on the forest, soil, and land. Apart from rudimentary cultivation practices, the Korkus are involved in practices like food-gathering, wine making, hunting and fishing as sub occupations. Due to the enactment of the Laws of Forest department and after the declaration of Melghat as a reserved forest for the protection of tigers, the Korkus have been experiencing severe restrictions, there is a strong sense of agitation amongst them as it has restricted their movements, shifting cultivation practices, grazing and hunting of wild animals. Though Project Tiger and Reserved Forests are important, it is necessary that government reviews its strategies as to whom to protect. On one hand are the constitutional rights of the scheduled tribes, that ensure them complete freedom to practice their traditional occupations and preservation of culture and at the same time are the abovementioned laws and rules that prevent them from undertaking a number of activities. Many of the residents explained about the disturbance they have been facing, as they are unable to protect their crop from wild animals and due to restrictions on hunting, they are not able to consume non-vegetarian food which was entirely procured from this activity.

Lack of Communication Facilities: An official from the Melghat Cell created in the DHO office, Amravati expressed that a lot of changes with regards to the attitude and response from the tribal have occurred in last ten years. However, there are some very basic administrative difficulties to be overcome like transportation and communication to these remote parts, as many times the facilities are not made available.

New Strategies for the Traditional Healers: Bhumkas, Bhagats and Padiyals as traditional healers of Melghat still continue to command a lot of confidence and demand from the tribal population. Earlier, they would not allow people to come to PHC and take medicines. However, the Public Health Department has come up with a bright idea since 1996-97, which comprises of catching up with these healers and training them for advising people as well as distributing some basic medicines like Paracetamol and Becosules in emergency. To some extent, this has definitely changed the attitudes of these healers.

Delay in Grants: The local officials at Semadoh PHC spoke about the bureaucratic delays in the arrival of grants for the beneficiaries in schemes like Matrutwa Anudan Yojana, wherein the beneficiaries lose their patience and fight with the health authorities for want of grants, however, it is very difficult to explain them that the grants have to be acquired from the BDO's office and further distributed. Most of the times the grant arrives when the woman has completed her last trimester of pregnancy and the provision of grants actually defeat its purpose.

Need for Enter-Education: The District Education Media Officer, Amravati, expressed that after working for a number of years with the Korku people, the experience has shown that the local *yatras* and *mahotsava* are the best platforms to extend IEC. Apart from this education through entertainment is the best media that has attracted attention from the Korkus.

IEC to be Looked at as a Process: One of the officials rightly pointed out that communication does not mean just one time awareness generation, but necessarily appropriate implementation of all the components of service delivery also amounts to effective communication. The availability of staff at PHC and Sub Center, catering to the patients in emergency situations and talking to the patients with concern also is a significant aspect of communication. This indicates that effective and impact oriented IEC thus emphasizes more on the humane approach and process of reaching out to the audience through various channels rather than focusing mainly upon the stereotyped channels like print and electronic media. The official also complained that every time any assessment of IEC in the state highlights only the work being done by the state IEC Bureau and the material prepared by it.[17]

REFERENCES

1. Interview of A. S. Shahade, the Deputy. C.E.O, Zilla Parishad, Amravati.

2. Interviews: The concerned officials have requested anonymity.

3. Interview of Dr. Subhash Salunke, Director General of Health Services, Public Health Department, Maharashtra State.

5. Interview of Dr. Subhash Salunke, n. 3.

6. *Ibid.*

7. Interview of Mr. Digvijay Khanvilkar, Health Minister, Maharashtra State.
8. Interview of Mr. Naveen Kumar, Principal Secretary, Public Health, Public Health Department, Maharashtra State.
9. Interview of Dr. Subhash Salunke, n. 3.
10. The officials who were interviewed expressed their desire not to be quoted by name.
11 The officials who were interviewed expressed their desire not to be quoted by name.
12. Interview of Dr. Subhash Salunke, n. 3.
13. Interview of Dr. Manmohan Singh, Principal Secretary, Family Welfare, Public Health Department, Maharashtra State.
14. Interview of Mr. Digvijay Khanvilkar, n. 7.
15. The officials who were interviewed expressed their desire not to be quoted by name.
16. The officials who were interviewed expressed their desire not to be quoted by name.
17. The officials who were interviewed expressed their desire not to be quoted by name.

8

Communication Strategies in a Tribal Community

A Case Study

Introduction

The present study attempts to analyze the impact of Public Health Policies related to Reproductive Health of women. Data has been collected from the couples in reproductive age from the Korku Community, which reflects their views regarding general health, Reproductive Health, Health Communication, the benefits received from various government schemes of Public Health Department.

The analysis presented here is a result of information collected from:

- Couples of reproductive age
- Couples receiving benefits of government schemes
- Employees of Primary Health Center

Couples of Reproductive Age

The following tables focus on:

(a) The profile of the couples in reproductive age;

(b) The information the couples possess with regards to health in general;

(c) The problems faced by the couples with regards to Reproductive Health in particular and their coping mechanisms;

(d) Information the couples have gathered through various communication agencies and strategies and

(e) Impact of these communication media felt by the couples.

(a) The Profile of the Couples

The profile here, means a representation of information by tables recorded in a quantified form. The profile in the present context is about the couples of reproductive age from fifteen villages of Semadoh Primary Health Center, Chikhaldara block of Amravati district. The first six tables give us a demographic profile of these couples related to age, educational level, caste, marital status, age of the husband and wife at the time of marriage, number of male and female members in the family, occupation, total income of the family, income from land and wages earned. The profile is the biographical sketch of these couples, which would give us an idea about the home situation. All these factors impinge on the well being of the women and the kind of care, support and inputs they get from their husbands and family members with regards to their reproductive health problems.

Age –Wise Distribution

Age as a factor in the present context is very important as the age of the couples determines their experience and understanding about the general and reproductive health issues.

Table 8.01

Showing Age-wise distribution of couples

Value label	*Frequency*	*Percentage*
18-25	88	44.0
26-35	57	28.5
36-45	40	20.0
46 and above	15	7.5
Grand Total	**200**	**100.0**

It would be seen from the data presented that the majority (44%) of the couples fall into the age group of 18-25 years. 28.5% of the couples fall in the age group of 26-35 years and 20% of the couples fall in the age group of 36-45 years. It is only 7.5% couples above the age of 46 years. This is indicative of the fact that almost all the couples fall in the reproductive age. Majority of the couples are in the age group 18-35, in the most crucial phase of building their families and rearing children as well as a potential period for facing reproductive health problems.

Education-wise Distribution

Educational qualification of the person determines the capacity to understand the socio-cultural and political aspects and helps develop the insights to tackle issues related to the same.

Table 8.02

Showing education wise distribution

Value label	*Frequency*	*Percentage*
Can not read or write	131	65.5
Can read only	35	17.5
Up to IV std	20	10.0
Up to X std	6	3.0
Up to XII std	8	4.0
Grand Total	**200**	**100.0**

It would be seen from the data presented that a majority (65.5%) of the couples do not have literacy status and cannot read or write. A sizeable number (17.5% + 10%) can manage to read and have studied up to 4th std. respectively. Very few couples have attained school education. The educational status of the couples definitely indicates their capacity and inclination towards understanding the print media as well as capacity to derive health education from the programs undertaken in order to extend an understanding on the aspects related to their health.

Caste Wise Distribution

The centuries old caste system is the criteria used by the Government to distribute the benefits of the schemes/programs initiated by it for the health of the women. The objective is to extend and improve maternal and child health services by targeting the weaker and backward sections of the society.

Table 8.03

Showing caste-wise distribution

Value label	*Frequency*	*Percentage*
Gond	7	3.5
Korku	193	96.5
Grand Total	**200**	**100.0**

It would be seen from data presented that majority of couples belong to Korku tribe and very few the Gond tribe as Melghat has Korkus in majority. Both Korkus and Gonds fall into the Constitutional list of Scheduled Tribes.

Marital Status-wise Distribution

Table 8.04

Showing marital status-wise distribution

Value label	*Frequency*	*Percentage*
Married	190	95.0
Widow	6	3.0
Not available	4	2.0
Grand Total	**200**	**100.0**

It would be seen from the data presented that 95% of the couples continue to have marital bonds, whereas 6 women are leading lives of widowhood. 4 women have not expressed about their marital status, as amongst the Korkus the women are allowed to live separately if they want to.

Wife's Age at the Time of Marriage

The wife's age at the time of marriage reflects her maturity and capacity to take proper decision regarding her life and her capability to start a family.

Table 8.05

Showing wife's age at the time of marriage

Value Label	*Frequency*	*Percentage*
15	3	1.5
16	47	23.5
17	47	23.5
18	72	36
19	21	10.5
20	10	5
Grand Total	**200**	**100**

It would be seen from the data presented that majority of the women got married at the age of 16 to 18, that is 83% where as only 15.5% have got married above the age of 18 years.

Husband's Age at the Time of Marriage

Similarly the husband's age at the time of marriage reflects her maturity and capacity to take proper decision regarding her life and her capability to start a family.

Table 8.06

Showing husband's age at time of marriage

Value Label	*Frequency*	*Percentage*
17	8	4.0
18	34	17.0
19	12	6.0
20	91	45.5
21	25	12.5
22	29	14.5
28	1	0.5
Grand Total	**200**	**100.0**

It would be seen from the data presented that most of the men, 85% men married in the age group of 17 to 21 and very few above i.e. 15% men after completing the age of 21 years.

Number of Members in the Family

Table 8.07

Showing number of members in the family

Value Label	*Frequency*	*Percentage*
1-4	21	10.5
5-7	113	56.5
More than 7	66	33
Grand Total	**200**	**100**

It would be seen from the data presented that majority of house holds, 56.5% have 5 to 7 members in the family, only 10 .5% families have four members each and about 33% of the families have more than 7 members. Hence average number of family members is between 5-7 or more than 7.

Number of Female Members in the Family

Table 8.08 a

Showing number of female members in the family

Value Label	*Frequency*	*Percentage*
1	19	9.5
2	66	33.0
3	76	38.0
4	19	9.5
5	10	5.0
6	8	4.0
8	2	1.0
Grand Total	**200**	**100.0**

It would be seen from the data presented that about 33% & 38% families have 2 and 3 female members respectively. There are few families that is, 19.5% of the families having more then 4 female members.

Number of Male Members in the Family

Table 8.08 b

Showing number of male members in the family

Value Label	*Frequency*	*Percentage*
0	2	1.0
1	28	14.0
2	50	25.0
3	69	34.5
4	29	14.5
5	18	9.0
6	4	2.0
Grand Total	**200**	**100.0**

It would be seen from the data presented that 49% of the families have 3 to 4 male members and about 11% 5 to 6 male members, 29% with just one or two male members and only two families do not have male members at all. Normally, amongst the Korkus and Gonds, they look forward to birth of a son and hence it would be seen that the number of male members is generally higher than the number of female members in the family.

Number of Children in the Family

Table 8.09 a

Showing number of children in the family

Number of Children	*Frequency*	*Percentage*
0	10	5.0
1	21	10.5
2	48	24.0
3	50	25.0
4	51	25.5
5	16	8.0
6	1	0.5
8	1	0.5
9	1	0.5
10	1	0.5
Grand Total	**200**	**100.0**

It would be seen from the data presented that most of the families have 1-4 children and only 10% of the families have 5-9 children. 10% families do not have children at all.

Son Preference

Table 8.09 b

Showing number of sons in the family

Number of children	*Frequency*
1	4
2	4
3	7
4	3
5	3
Grand Total	**21**

Occupation Wise Distribution

Table 8.10

Showing occupation wise distribution

Value Label	*Frequency*	*Percentage*
Chowkidar & labourer	2	1.0
Compounder	1	0.5
Farming and labourer	177	88.5
Labourer	15	7.5
Dai	1	0.5
Helper-phc	1	0.5
Kotwal	1	0.5
Sarpanch , Lipik	1	0.5
Social worker/labourer	1	0.5
Total	**200**	**100.0**

It would be seen from the data presented that majority, 88.5% of the families are involved in farming and also work as labourers. About 7.5% of the families work only as labourers as they don't have land for farming. Very few families have occupations like chowkidar, compounder, helper, dai, surpanch etc.

Total Income of the Family

Table 8.11

Showing total income of the family

Value Label	*Frequency*	*Percentage*
Less than 1500	146	73.0
1501-2500	38	19.0
2501-5000	15	7.5
More than 5000	1	0.5
Grand Total	**200**	**100.0**

It would be seen from the data presented that majority (73%) of the families have less then 1500 Rs./month as income for the entire family. 19% of the families earn between Rs1500 & 2500. 7.5% families earn between Rs. 2500 & 5000 and just one family earns more than Rs. 5000/month.

Subsidiary Occupations of the Families

Table 8.12

Showing Subsidiary occupations of the families

Value Label	*Frequency*	*Percentage*
Food gathering, hunting, wine making and fishing	200	100.0
Grand Total	**200**	**100.0**

100% families practice food-gathering, wine making, hunting and fishing as sub occupations.

Income from Land

Table 8.13

Showing income from land

Value Label	*Frequency*	*Percentage*
Jowar	7	3.5
Jowar and tur	4	2.0
Rice and tur	60	30.0
Rice production	62	31.0
Tur and jowar	48	24.0
Not practicing agriculture	19	9.5
Grand Total	**200**	**100.0**

It would be seen from the data presented that majority (61%) are yielding rice & tur production. Whereas, 24% of take the yield of tur & jowar. 9.5% families do not practice agriculture.

Daily Wages

Table 8.14

Showing daily wages

Value Label	*Frequency*	*Percentage*
30-40	171	85.5
30-45	2	1.0
35-45	7	3.5
40-45	1	0.5
Not Working on daily wages	19	9.5
Grand Total	**200**	**100.0**

It would be seen from the data presented that 85.5% of the families draw their daily wages between Rs. 30-40 per day. Very few families that is 14.5% are able to earn wages more then Rs. 40Rs per day.

(b) The information the couples possess with regards to health in general

Immunization of Children

Table 8.15

Showing whether the children are taken for immunization

Value Label	*Frequency*	*Percentage*
Yes	200	100.0
No	0	0.0
Total	**200**	**100.0**

100% people take their children for immunization.

Approach during Illness

Table 8.16

Showing where do they go in case of any kind of illness

Value Label	*Frequency*	*Percentage*
ANM	43	21.5
Bhumka	31	15.5
Doctor	80	40.0
Doctor, Bhagat/Bhumka	46	23.0
Grand Total	**200**	**100.0**

It would be seen from the data presented that 40% of the families approach the PHC Dctor in case of illness, 21.5% approach the ANM and 15.5% approach the traditional healer Bhumka/Padiyal. About 23% families approach the Doctor as well as Bhumka at the same time. The data indicates that people still have belief in the traditional healers and their methods of treatments for illnesses.

Satisfaction with the Services Received

Table 8.17

Showing whether they are happy with the services received at the time of illness

Value Label	*Frequency*	*Percentage*
No	76	38.0
Yes	124	62.0
Grand Total	**200**	**100.0**

It would be seen from the data presented that 62% of the couples have expressed satisfaction regarding the services that they receive at the time of illness be it doctor ANM, Bhumka or Padiyal. However, 38% of the couples have expressed unhappiness regarding the services received.

Deaths of Children-0-5 Years

Table 8.18 a

Showing deaths of children in the family for last three years of age group 0 to 5 years.

Value Label	*Frequency*	*Percentage*
None	167	83.5
1	23	11.5
2	5	2.5
3	3	1.5
4	1	0.5
6	1	0.5
Grand Total	**200**	**100.0**

It would be seen from the data presented that 16.5% of the couples have lost their children in the age group of 0-5 years in last three years, the number varying from 1-6. This indicates that infant mortality is still continuing to accrue in tribal families of Melghat.

Causes of Deaths

Table 8.18 b

Showing causes of deaths

Value Label	*Frequency*	*Percentage*
Do not know-may be illness	1	3.03
Illness	19	57.58
Illness and diarrhoea	1	3.03
Illness and weakness	6	18.18
Illness, weakness and malnutrition	1	3.03
Lather in the mouth-6 days old	1	3.03
Malnutrition	1	3.03
Still birth	1	3.03
Weakness by birth	2	6.06
Grand Total	**33**	**100.00**

It would be seen from the data presented that out of total 33 children who have lost their lives in infancy about 57.58 have died due to general illness, while others have mention about diarrhea and weakness. Incase of one child it is mentioned as malnutrition. Again in case of another child he is said to have died due to lather in the mouth and one child was still born. In case of one child the parents do not know the cause of death.

Special Care during Pregnancy

Table 8.19

Showing special care taken during pregnancy

Value Label	*Frequency*	*Percentage*
Provide regular food	200	100.0
Total	**200**	**100.0**

It would be seen from the data presented that 100% people responded that no special care is taken during pregnancy but regular food is provided.

Nutritional Care during Pregnancy

Table 8.20

Showing special food/nutrition provided to the pregnant woman

Value Label	*Frequency*	*Percentage*
Bayal, gugudu-like potato	17	8.5
Chana	1	0.5
Chana, kutki and ghee	38	19.0
Kutki and soyabean	1	0.5
Kutki, ghee	2	1.0
Kutki, ghee and rice	51	25.5
Roasted mahua	42	21.0
Soyabean	1	0.5
Soyabean and kutki	47	23.5
Grand Total	**200**	**100.0**

It would be seen from the data presented that the most common special food/nutrition provided to the pregnant women is kutki, ghee and soyabean where as some other products like bayal, gugudu, chana, roasted mahua, and rice is also given as nutritious food.

Care to Increase the Quantity of Breast Milk

Table 8.21

Showing food consumed by new mothers to increase the quantity of breast milk

Value Label	*Frequency*	*Percentage*
Kutki, ghee and milk	52	26.0
Kutki and ghee	79	39.5
Kutki, Dal and roti	69	34.5
Grand Total	**200**	**100.0**

It would be seen from the data presented that 39.5% women consume kutki and ghee to increase the quantity of breast milk. 34.5% have expressed a combination of kutki dal and roti, and 26% have expressed kutki ghee and milk as nutrition for the same, however it must be noted that kutki is one of the most popular and easily available nutritional food.

Instrument Used to cut the Umbilical Cord

Table 8.22 a

Showing the instrument used to cut the umbilical cord

Value Label	*Frequency*	*Percentage*
Blade	146	73.0
Scissor	52	26.0
Stone	2	1.0
Grand Total	**200**	**100.0**

It would be seen from the data presented that 73% of the couples responded that a blade is used to cut the umbilical cord whereas 26% talked about using a scissor. Only one couple mentioned about stone as the cutting instrument.

Sterilization of Instrument before Cutting

Table 8.22 b

Showing whether the instrument is sterilized before use

Value Label	*Frequency*	*Percentage*
Yes	139	69.5
Do Not know	61	30.5
Grand Total	**200**	**100**

It would be seen from the data presented that 69.5% couples are aware of the sterilization process of the cutting instruments whereas 30.5% couples did know about this process.

Special Care of the Child Immediately after Birth

Table 8.23 a

Showing special care taken of the child immediately after birth

Value Label	*Frequency*	*Percentage*
Some times the child is given goat milk	14	7.0
Sometimes mother has no milk so cow milk is given	21	10.5
The child is cleaned and immediately given colostrum milk	48	24.0
The child is given milk after few hours of delivery	60	30.0
The child is given milk the next day after delivery	38	19.0
The child is given mothers milk after three days	19	9.5
Grand Total	**200**	**100.0**

It would be seen from the data presented that only 24% of the women clean the child and immediately feed colostrum milk, whereas 30% have expressed that any kind of milk is given to the child after few hours of delivery. About 7% & 10.5% couples have responded that the child is given either goat milk or cow milk respectively in cases the mother has no milk. 19% of the women expressed that the child is fed with milk only on the next day of the delivery and 9.5% have expressed that the mother's milk is fed after three days of the delivery. It is important to note that about 28.5% families still think that the new-born child should not be fed with milk immediately after birth and wait for one or three days.

Feeding of Colostrum Milk

Table 8.23 b

Showing whether the mother feeds the child colostrum milk

Value Label	*Frequency*	*Percentage*
No	57	28.5
Yes	143	71.5
Grand Total	**200**	**100.0**

It would be seen from the data presented that 71.5% of mothers feed colostrum milk to the child, whereas remaining 28.5% do not prefer to feed the colostrum milk.

Feeding Water to the Child

Table 8.24 a

Showing whether the mother gives water to infant

Value Label	*Frequency*	*Percentage*
No	126	63.0
Yes	74	37.0
Grand Total	**200**	**100.0**

It would be seen from the data presented that 63.0% of the couples do not prefer to feed the child with water and only 37% prefer to feed the water to the new born child.

Duration of feeding of water to the infants

Table 8.24 b

Showing number of days water is not given to infant

Value Label	*Frequency*	*Percentage*
2 months	45	35.71
40 days	51	40.48
For 3 months	30	23.81
Grand Total	**126**	**100.00**

It would be seen from the data presented that majority (40.48%) do not feed the child with water for almost 40 days, whereas 35.71% couples feed the water after 2 months of period and 23.81% feed water after a period 3 months.

Breast Feeding to the Child

Table 8.25

Showing whether breast feeding to a child starts immediately after the birth

Value Label	*Frequency*	*Percentage*	*Reason*
No	57	28.5	The initial milk is not good for the baby
Yes	143	71.5	
Grand Total	**200**	**100**	

It would be seen from the data presented that 71.5% women start breast feeding immediately after the birth of the child where as 28.5% have expressed that the initial milk of the mother is not good for the baby and hence breast feeding should not start immediately after the child's birth.

Conducting of Deliveries

Table 8.26

Showing who conducts the delivery of a woman

Value Label	*Frequency*	*Percentage*
Dai	136	68.0
Doctor	64	32.0
Grand Total	**200**	**100.0**

It would be seen from the data presented that 68% of the deliveries are conducted by the local Dai & are not institutional deliveries where as only 32% are conducted at the hospital (institutional deliveries) by the doctor.

Remuneration for Dai

Table 8.26 b

Showing what the dai receives in return for the service she renders

Value Label	*Frequency*	*Percentage*
100 Rs	44	32.35
100 Rs. and a saree	55	40.44
50 Rs.	37	27.21
Grand Total	**136**	**100.00**

It would be seen from the data presented that 40.44% of the couples pay Rs. 100 and sari to the Dai who conducts the delivery where as 32.35% and 27.21% pay Rs. 100 and Rs. 50 for the task respectively.

Umbilical Cord

Table 8.27

Showing what is done with the umbilical cord

Value Label	*Frequency*	*Percentage*
Buried after five days	200	100.0
Total	**200**	**100.0**

It would be seen from the data presented that 100% people said Umbilical Cord is buried after 5 days.

Rituals and Ceremonies Associated with the Birth of Child

Table 8.28

Showing the various rituals/ceremonies associated with the birth of girl/boy child

Value Label	*Frequency*	*Percentage*
5th Day, 12th Day, Dai Pooja	200	100.0
Grand Total	**200**	**100.0**

It would be seen from the data presented that 100% couples responded that they perform "5th day, 12th day and Dai Pooja"

Rest for the New Mother

Table 8.29

Showing how long does the new mother rests before she starts her daily routine

Value Label	*Frequency*	*Percentage*
40 days	114	57.0
60 days	86	43.0
Grand Total	**200**	**100.0**

It would be seen from the data that 57% of the couples expressed that 40 days is the general rest period for the mother after the delivery, whereas 43% expressed 60 days as the rest period.

Medication during Prenatal Period

Table 8.30 a

Showing the medication a midwife provides for the new mother during prenatal period

Value Label	*Frequency*	*Percentage*
Iron tablets	163	81.5
No knowledge	37	18.5
Grand Total	**200**	**100**

It would be seen from the data presented that 81.5% women are aware of and consume iron tablets as medicine in prenatal period, whereas 18.5% express that they have no knowledge about any kind of medicine during prenatal period.

Medication during Postnatal Period

Table 8.30 b

Showing the medication a midwife provides for the new mother during postnatal period

Value Label	*Frequency*	*Percentage*
No medicines	200	100.0
Total	**200**	**100.0**

It would be seen from the data presented that 100% couples responded that they do not take any medicine in the post-natal period.

Duration of Breast Feeding

Table 8.31

Showing how many months/years the child is breast fed

Value Label	*Frequency*	*Percentage*
1 year	77	38.5
2 years	90	45.0
6 months	33	16.5
Grand Total	**200**	**100.0**

It would be seen from the data presented that majority (45%) of the couples expressed that the child is breast fed for almost two years. 38.5% & 16.5% couples expressed breast feeding period as one year and six months respectively.

Weaning Foods for the Child

Table 8.32 a

Showing which age weaning foods are given to a child

Value Label	*Frequency*	*Percentage*
12 months	32	16.0
4 months	40	20.0
6 months	128	64.0
Grand Total	**200**	**100.0**

It would be seen from the data presented that majority (64%) of the couples start the weaning food as soon as 6 months are completed. 20% & 16% couples expressed 4 months and 12 months as the starting time respectively.

Types of Weaning Foods

Table 8.32 b

Showing which weaning foods are given to a child

Value Label	*Frequency*	*Percentage*
Cow milk, dal and rice	1	0.5
Dal and rice	29	14.5
Rice kheer, dal and rice	11	5.5
Rice water	80	40
Tur dal water	79	39.5
Grand Total	**200**	**100**

It would be seen from the data presented that majority (40 & 39.5%) of couples give rice water & tur dal water as weaning foods respectively. 14.5% couples give a combination of dal & rice, whereas 0.5% also give cow milk as weaning food.

Reporting during Epidemic

Table 8.33

Showing who reports to the government in case of epidemic

Value Label	*Frequency*	*Percentage*
Traditional Dai/healer and Medical Officer	39	19.5
Traditional Dai/healer, Medical Officer, A.N.M./LHV	1	0.5
Traditional Dai/healer and Medical Officer Private Doctor /clinic	56	28.0
Medical Officer and Drug Store	48	24.0
Private Doctor /clinic and others	56	28.0
Grand Total	**200**	**100.0**

It would be seen from the data presented that 28% of the families expressed that the private doctor, Dai, Bhumka or Medical Officer informs the government in case of epidemic. 28% also said that it is only the private doctors who informs. 24% said that either Medical Officer or the drug store informs the Govt.

(c) Problems Faced by the Couples with Regards to Reproductive Health in Particular and Their Coping Mechanisms

Reproductive Health Problems

Table 8.34 a

Showing the reproductive health problems faced

Value Label	*Frequency*	*Percentage*
No Problems	11	5.50
Frequency of children/less periods/ menstrual problems	26	13.00
Abdominal pains/backache	75	37.50
White discharge	65	32.50
Vaginal irritation/infection	36	18.00
Frequent and irregular periods	26	13.00
Stomach ache	20	10.00
Menopause	1	0.50
Cancerous tumor/continuous irritation	2	1.00
Tubectomy failed/ irritation/pregnancy	5	2.50

It would be seen from the data presented that 37.5% of women face abdominal pains and back ache, 32.5% suffer from white discharge, 18% suffer from vaginal irritation and infection, 13% from menstrual problems, 13% from frequent and irregular periods and 10% from stomach ache. 5.5% of women expressed that they do not face any reproductive health problems. Some women complained of cancerous tumor, failure of tubectomy and menopause. It is important to note that women took a lot of time to express their reproductive health problems, and did not mention anything related to natural or unnatural abortions unless asked specifically.

Table 8.34 b

Showing the RH problems faced specifically related to natural/unnatural abortions

Value Label	*Frequency*	*Percentage*
Yes	83	41.5
No	117	58.5
Total	**200**	**100.0**

It would be seen from the data presented that apart from the various problems mentioned regarding reproductive health, which the women faced on a day to day basis, 41.5% of the women talked about the facing problems due to natural or unnatural abortions.

Approach during the Reproductive Health Problem

Table 8.35

Showing whom women approach during any reproductive health problem

Value label	*Frequency*	*Percentage*
ANM	18	9.0
Bhumka	18	9.0
Dai or ANM	83	41.5
LHV or ANM	50	25.0
PHC	24	12.0
PHC or even rural hospital	7	3.5
Grand Total	**200**	**100.0**

It would be seen from the data presented that 41.5% of women approach the Dai or ANM, 25% approach the LHV or ANM, 12% approach the PHC, 9% approach only the ANM and 9% approach the traditional healer bhumka in case of any reproductive health problem. Only 3.5% women expressed about approaching rural hospital, these were also the women who can afford to go a long distance.

Information Regarding Remedies

Table 8.36

Showing who has informed regarding the remedies?

Value label	*Frequency*	*Percentage*
ANM	99	49.5
Bhumka	18	9
Dai	83	41.5
Grand Total	**200**	**100**

It would be seen from the data presented that 49.5% of women are informed regarding the remedies for reproductive health problems by ANM, 41.5% are informed by the Dai & 9% are informed by bhumka.

Home-based Care for Reproductive Health Problems

Table 8.37

Showing what home based care is taken to cope up with the reproductive health problems

Value label	*Frequency*	*Percentage*
Application of oils	15	7.5
Not aware of any home-based remedy	27	13.5
Nothing as such	50	25
Roasted Mahua flowers	49	24.5
Some herbal leaves or drinks	35	17.5
Tying up bark of the tree around the waist	24	12
Grand Total	**200**	**100**

It would be seen from the data presented that 24.5% women consume roasted mahua flowers, 17.5% consume herbal leaves or drinks, 12% tie a bark of the tree around the waist, 7.5% apply different types of oils, as remedies for reproductive health problems. 13.5% women express that they do not know of any remedy and 25% express that they do not go for any remedy and suffer as it is.

Participation in the Programs on Reproductive Health

Table 8.38

Showing whether the couples have participated in any of the information sharing program on reproductive health undertaken by the government in the village

Value label	*Frequency*	*Percentage*
No	29	14.5
Yes	171	85.5
Grand Total	**200**	**100**

It would be seen from the data presented that 85.5% couples expressed that they have participated information sharing program on reproductive health where as 14.5% couples said they have never participated in any such program.

Ideal Number of Children

Table 8.39

Showing what according to the couples is the ideal number of children you should have

Value label	*Frequency*	*Percentage*
2	121	60.5
3	77	38.5
4	2	1
Grand Total	**200**	**100**

It would be seen from the data presented that 60.5% couple feel that having two children is ideal where as 38.5% couples feel 3 is the ideal number. Only 1% of couple have express 4 is the ideal number.

Awareness of Family Planning Methods

Table 8.40 a

Showing awareness regarding family planning methods

Value label	*Frequency*	*Percentage*
Yes	200	100.0
Total	**200**	**100.0**

It would be seen from the data presented that 100% of the couples responded that they are aware of Family Planning Methods.

Awareness of Benefits of Family Planning Methods

Table 8.40 b

Showing awareness of the benefits of the family planning

Value label	*Frequency*	*Percentage*
Yes	200	100.0
Total	**200**	**100.0**

It would be seen from the data presented that 100% of the couples responded that they are aware of the benefits of the Family Planning Methods.

Procurement of Information Regarding Family Planning

Table 8.41

Showing who has informed the couples regarding family planning

Value label	*Frequency*	*Percentage*
ANM	56	28
Dai	26	13
Gram Sevak	20	10
LHV	33	16.5
Patwari	29	14.5
PHC Doctor	21	10.5
Sarpanch	15	7.5
Grand Total	**200**	**100**

It would be seen from the data presented that 28% of the couples have been informed about Family Planning by the ANM, 16.5% by the LHV, 14.5% by the Patwari, 13% by the Dai, 10.5% by the PHC Doctor, 10% by the Gram Sevak and 7.5% by the Sarpanch. Thus, it shows that it is several people in the village who generally inform the villagers about this.

Awareness Regarding Different Methods of Family Planning

Table 8.42

Showing what other methods the couples are aware of

Value label	*Frequency*	*Percentage*
Condoms and pills	53	26.5
Tubectomy and pills	81	40.5
Vasectomy, laproscopy	66	33
Grand Total	**200**	**100**

It would be seen from the data presented that 40.5% couples are aware of tubectomy and pills, 33% are aware of vasectomy and laproscopy, 26.5% are aware of condoms and pills as the different methods of Family Planning.

Contraceptive Methods Used

Table 8.43

Showing what contraceptive measure couples are using

Value label	*Frequency*	*Percentage*
Condoms	9	4.5
Tubectomy	41	20.5
Not using	86	43
Infertility	2	1
Laproscopy	1	0.5
Pills	42	21
Traditional medicine	1	0.5
Vasectomy	18	9
Grand Total	**200**	**100**

It would be seen from the data presented that 43% of the couples have not adopted any contraceptive measures. Amongst the remaining 57% couples, 20% couples have adopted tubectomy, 21% women are using pills, 9% have under gone vasectomy, 4.5% are using condoms, 0.5% are using traditional medicine, 0.5% have undergone laproscopy and only 1% couples are suffering from infertility.

Traditional Contraceptives

Table 8.44

Showing whether any traditional contraceptive methods are used

Value Label	*Frequency*	*Percentage*
N	182	91
Y	18	9
Grand Total	**200**	**100**

It would be seen from the data presented that 91% of couples have said that they are not using any traditional contraceptive methods and only 9% have expressed that they are using some kind of traditional contraceptive methods.

Provision of Contraceptives

Table 8.45

Showing who provides you with the contraceptives

Value Label	*Frequency*	*Percentage*
ANM	7	3.5
PHC staff/ANM	51	25.5
N.A.	142	71
Grand Total	**200**	**100**

It would be seen from the data presented that 71% have expressed that they are not provided with any kind of contraceptives by any body. 25.5% have expressed that they are provided with contraceptives by either PHC staff or ANM where as only 3.5% said that ANM is the exclusive provider of contraceptives.

(d) Information the Couples have Gathered Through various communication agencies and strategies

Sources of Communication

Table 8.46

Showing the general sources of communication regarding reproductive health

Value label	*Frequency*	*Percentage*
Television, Radio, Street plays, Posters	6	3.0
Radio, Plays, Street plays, Health workers	32	16.0
Radio, Plays, Street plays, Health workers, Posters	76	38.0
Radio, Street plays, Health workers	38	19.0
Radio, Street plays, Health workers, NGOs	1	0.5
NGOs, Health workers, Posters	47	23.5
Grand Total	**200**	**100.0**

It would be seen from the data presented that 38% couples have mentioned radio, plays, street plays, health workers and posters as general sources of communication regarding reproductive health. 23.5% have mentioned NGOs health workers and posters; 16% have mentioned radio plays street plays and health workers; 19% have mentioned radio street plays and health workers; 3% have mention TV, radio, street plays and posters; and 0.5% have mentioned radio, street plays, health workers, NGOs as general sources of communication.

It would be seen from the data presented that 51% of couples have mentioned about ANMs, PHC staff and health workers as the agencies of communication. 19% have mentioned ANMs, PHC staff, NGOs and health workers; 8.5% have mentioned PHC doctors, ANM, PHC staff and health workers; and 4% have mentioned government officials, NGOs, health workers as the different agencies of communications. 17.5% couples have said that they do not know of any agencies of communication.

Health Education Agencies

Table 8.47

Showing health education agencies/communicators

Value Label	*Frequency*	*Percentage*
PHC Doctors ANMs/PHC staff Health workers	17	8.5
ANMs/PHC staff Health workers	102	51
ANMs/PHC staff NGOs Health workers	38	19
Government officials NGOs Health workers	8	4
None as such	35	17.5
Grand Total	**200**	**100**

Understanding from the Sources

Table 8.48

Showing understanding from these communication sources

Value Label	*Frequency*	*Percentage*
Abortions should be avoided for better health, less pregnancies are important for good health	2	1
Family planning is necessary to have a small family, good nutrition is necessary	36	18
Hygiene and cleanliness is important	29	14.5
Less pregnancies are important for good health	32	16
The ANM says, there is more to our health than just bearing children	21	10.5
The daughters should be married after 18 years of age	32	16
The daughters should be married after 18 years of age, abortions should be avoided	1	0.5
The delivery should take place in the hospital	16	8
The health workers and ANM give us good information	2	1
Women should have good nutrition to have a healthy baby	29	14.5
Grand Total	**200**	**100**

It would be seen from the data presented that 18% of the couples have understood that Family Planning is necessary as well as good nutrition should be followed.14.5% couples have understood about the necessity of good nutrition for women in order to have healthy baby. 14.5% of couples understood regarding hygiene and cleanliness. 10.5% have expressed that it is more important to look after ones health rather than just bearing children. 8% have understood the importance of institutional delivery. 16% have understood the importance of less pregnancy for good health. 16% have expressed that the daughter should be married after the 18 yrs. of age. 1% have expressed about receiving good information from health workers and ANM. And 0.5% have felt that abortion should be avoided.

Language of the Communication Media

Table 8.49

Showing whether the couples are comfortable with the language of communication media

Value Label	*Frequency*	*Percentage*
Mostly	15	7.5
Not always	58	29
Not very comfortable	112	56
Sometimes	15	7.5
Grand Total	**200**	**100**

It would be seen from the data presented that 56% of the couples are not very comfortable about the language used by the media. 29% of the couples expressed that not always do they understand the language used. 7.5% have expressed that some times they are comfortable with the language. Only 7.5% couples expressed that they mostly understand every thing.

Requirement of Explanation – if – Lack of Understanding

Table 8.50

Showing whether the couples have asked for explanation in case of lack of understanding

Value Label	*Frequency*	*Percentage*
No	120	60
Yes	80	40
Grand Total	**200**	**100**

It would be seen from the data presented that 60% of the couple have never asked for any kind of explanation in case of lack of understanding where as 40% of the couples have attempted to ask for clarifications.

Information Provision at Home

Table 8.51

Showing if the couples receive any information at home

Value Label	*Frequency*	*Percentage*
No	30	15
Yes	170	85
Grand Total	**200**	**100**

It would be seen from the data presented that 85% of the couples do receive some information at home where as 15% of the couples replied that they don't receive any information from home.

It would be seen from the data presented that 21% of the couples replied negatively that they don't receive any information when they go to the clinic or any other place. 17.5% couples spoke about information regarding hygiene and cleanliness; 17% spoke regarding contraception; 17% spoke regarding care during illness; 11% spoke regarding nutrition; 8.5% spoke regarding child care; and 8% spoke regarding drinking of boiled water.

Information at Clinics

Table 8.52

Showing what information the couples get when they go to the clinic or any other place

Value Label	*Frequency*	*Percentage*
None	42	21
Regarding care during illness	34	17
Regarding child care	17	8.5
Regarding contraception	34	17
Regarding drinking of boiled water	16	8
Regarding hygiene and cleanliness	35	17.5
Regarding nutrition	22	11
Grand Total	**200**	**100**

(e) Impact of these Communication Media Felt by the Couples

Knowledge Gained

Table 8.53

Showing the knowledge gained from these communicators

Value Label	*Frequency*	*Percentage*
None	42	21
Regarding care during illness	34	17
Regarding child care	17	8.5
Regarding contraception	34	17
Regarding drinking of boiled water	16	8
Regarding hygiene and cleanliness	35	17.5
Regarding nutrition	22.	11
Grand Total	**200**	**100**

It would be seen from the data presented that 21% of couples have expressed that they have not gained any knowledge form these communicators. Further, 17.5% couples expressed about hygiene and cleanliness; 17% regarding care during illness; 17% regarding contraception; 11% regarding nutrition; 8.5% regarding child care; and 8% couples expressed regarding knowledge about drinking of boiled water.

Adequacy of Sources of Communication

Table 8.54

Showing whether these sources for communication are enough

Value Label	*Frequency*	*Percentage*
The doctors should tell us about more options, how to overcome our RH problems	33	16.5
The entire responsibility of birth control is on us and the men refuse to use anything	34	17
The government facilities should be provided properly	35	17.5
The males of our families need to be convinced about the various problems that we suffer from	21	10.5
We cannot read and write, we need more explanation	77	38.5
Grand Total	**200**	**100**

It would be seen from the data presented that 38.5% couples expressed that they cannot read and write and hence need more explanation. 17.5% couples demanded that the government facilities should be provided properly. 17% couples expressed that the entire responsibility of birth control is shouldered on women and men refuse to use any contraceptive measures. 16.5% of the women expressed that doctors should give them more options and remedies to over come reproductive health problems. 10.5% of women have said that the men should be made aware of reproductive health problems faced by women.

Adequacy of Information Provided

Table 8.55

Showing whether the couples still need more information on their health

Value Label	*Frequency*	*Percentage*
No	0	0
Yes	200	100.0
Grand Total	**200**	**100.0**

It would be seen from the data presented that 100% couples expressed regarding the need for more information on health.

Opinion about Existing Medical and Health Services

Table 8.56

Showing what do the couples think about the existing medical and health services

Value Label	*Frequency*	*Percentage*
Despite operation I conceived again-what do I do	3	1.5
I feel there is corruption in this system and it needs be looked into	22	11
Many times it is out of our reach, the distance is too long	59	29.5
Most of the times, in emergency the people are not available	21	10.5
Refused for my tubectomy-they tell me your health is not good but I know-their quota is complete	4	2
The ANM / the LHV / the MPW are very helpful	44	22
We feel that the dai is better than the doctor	47	23.5
Grand Total	**200**	**100**

It would be seen from the data presented that 29.5% couples expressed that the medical facilities many times out of there reach and the distance is too long. 23.5% expressed that the Dai is the better then the doctor. 22% couples appreciated the helpful nature of ANM, LHVs and MPW. 11% couples complained about corruption in the system and demanded enquiry. 10.5% couples complained about lack of availability of PHC people in case of emergency. 2% couples complained about the authorities refusing to conduct tubectomy & also expressed that they do so because their quota is completed. 1.5% couples complaints about the failure of tubectomy.

Suggestion for Better Communication

Table 8.57

Do you have any suggestions for better communication with you

Value label	*Frequency*	*Percentage*
The ANM should have group and individual talks with us	29	14.5
The ANM should understand our problem	31	15.5
The doctor should be available for talking to us	32	16.0
The doctor should ensure us some guarantee regarding the operations undertaken	5	2.5
The facilities should be nearer to us	25	12.5
There should be people to talk to our men in the house	78	39.0
Grand Total	**200**	**100.0**

It would be seen from the data presented that 39% of the women suggested that the communicator should talk to the men in the family rather then just the women. 16% of the couples suggested that the doctors should be available at PHC to talk to us. 15.5% women demanded that ANM should under stand our problems. 14.5% suggested that ANM should have group and individual discussions with us. 12.5% suggested that health facility should be nearer to us. 2.5% couples suggested that the doctor should ensure some guarantee of the operations conducted.

Suggestions to State or Central Government

Table 8.58

Showing couples suggesting strategies for better communication to the state/central government

Value Label	*Frequency*	*Percentage*
Our problems are multifaceted, include health, environment, rights and many more things, the laws should be favourable	18	9
Same as earlier suggestion	163	81.5
The system has to favor the poor tribal and not exploit him/her	19	9.5
Grand Total	**200**	**100**

It would be seen from the data presented that 9% of the couples suggested that the problems of tribal people are multifaceted, which includes problems related to health, environmental rights, and the laws should favour them. 9.5% of the couples suggested that governmental system has to favour the poor tribals and not exploit them. 81.5% couples repeated their suggestions that are presented in the earlier table.

Changes in Attitude and Behaviour

Table 8.59

Showing whether any changes have taken place in personal attitude/ behaviour or family's attitude/behaviour towards health of women

Value Label	*Frequency*	*Percentage*
A lot of things are accepted-but still having a son is necessary-so no change	57	28.5
Both boys and girls are equal	15	7.5
Going to doctor and taking proper treatment is necessary	1	0.5
Health care is important	37	18.5
Lesser children is better	45	22.5
Marriage at a late age is a proper decision	28	14
Not really	17	8.5
Grand Total	**200**	**100**

It would be seen from the data presented that 28.5% couples expressed that our community has accepted a lot of new messages but having a son is still considered to be necessary and hence there appears to be no change in the behaviour. 22.5% of the couples expressed that it is better to have lesser children. 18.5% couples expressed that they have understood the importance of health care. 14% of couples said, they have accepted that marriage at a late age is a proper decision. 7.5% considered boys and girls as equal. 0.5% expressed about approaching doctor for proper treatment as a necessity step. However 8.5% couples felt that there has been no change in the attitudes and behaviour of people in the community.

The Impact Analysis of New Policies Implemented After the 1993 Crisis

Couples receiving Benefits of Government Schemes

Out of the 200 couples interviewed, 87 couples have received the benefits of various schemes specifically regarding reproductive health and also benefits from schemes of other departments. Though the focus is on the schemes from Public Health Department, the beneficiaries have spoken about the other schemes and provisions also.

The following tables focus on: Awareness and perception of government schemes in general and the ones meant for Reproductive Health of women; Information extended about the scheme; The infrastructural facility related to health available in the village; The usefulness of government schemes and the interest in knowing about them; The conduciveness of village environment to use the health facilities; The schemes the people have benefited from; The actual benefits received; The adequacy of the scheme; The difficulties faced in getting the scheme; The people approached in getting the benefits of the schemes; The response received from the higher officials to the difficulties presented by the couples; The visits of higher officials to the village; and the satisfaction experienced by the couples with the service provided by the government.

Awareness Regarding Government Schemes

Table 8.60

Showing the awareness regarding government schemes

Value label	*Frequency*	*Percentage*
Employment Guarantee Scheme	25	28.74
Matrutva Anudan Yojana	58	66.67
School facilities / Ashram school	18	20.69
Live stock farming	6	6.90
Dai scheme	8	9.20
Family planning incentive	5	5.75
Immunization	23	26.44
Agriculture: seed distribution	8	9.20
Water purification	13	14.94
Huts for Adivasis	20	22.99
Anganwadi	29	33.33
Padha swayam sevak scheme	3	3.45
Chulha Gas scheme	5	5.75
Yearly food grains for BPL	19	21.84
Mahila Mandal and bachat gat	3	3.45
Doctor scheme; monsoon	2	2.30
Supply of occupational equipments	4	4.60
Health education program	1	1.15

It would be seen from the data presented that majority (66.67%) of the couples have spoken about Matrutva Anudan Yojana, which is a combination of cash grants, grants for medicine and food allowance. Couples have also talked about the benefits derived from the Anganwadi scheme (33.3%) wherein they receive the nutritious food during pregnancy and in the period when they are nursing mothers. A number of other schemes have been mentioned which are meant for employment generation, education, savings and credit activities, education and health. Only 1 couple has mentioned regarding Health Education as a scheme of the government.

Perceptions Regarding Government Schemes

Table 8.61

Showing perception regarding government schemes

Value label	*Frequency*	*Percentage*
MAY money utilized for other purpose in the family	3	3.45
Development schemes are good	44	50.57
Information regarding schemes not available	17	19.54
Govt. gives more importance to forest/ tiger project/ animal	8	9.20
Confused	2	2.30
Benefits do not reach people/misused	38	43.68
Inadequate and limited benefits	10	11.49

It would be seen from the data presented that 50.57% couples have said that the development schemes are good, whereas 43.68% have expressed that the benefits do not reach people and are the schemes are misused. 19.54% couples expressed that the information regarding the schemes are not available; 11.49% expressed that the benefits provided are inadequate and limited; 9.20% expressed that government gives more importance to the forest, tiger project and animals and hence they are on a lower priority; 3.45% couples expressed that the MAY money is used for other purposes and is not really utilized for the pregnant mother; and 2.30% couples were confused about their perceptions.

It would be seen from the data presented that majority (86.21%) couples talked about the availability of PHC and Sub-center by the government and the specific scheme Matrutva Anudan Yojana provided for the pregnant and nursing mothers. 29.89 spoke about Anganwadi-diet scheme; 25.29 spoke of immunization for mothers during pregnancy; 10.34 spoke about the dai baithak yojana wherein the dais are trained by the medical professionals; 5.75% each spoke about sanitation programs and health check-up camps; 2.30% spoke about Padha Swayam Sewak scheme, wherein the padha workers from the village are trained for health education purpose. Whereas, 9.20% couples said that they were not aware of any schemes related to reproductive health of women.

Specific Schemes for Reproductive Health of Women

Table 8.62

Showing whether the beneficiaries know of any scheme specifically meant for reproductive health of women

Value label	*Frequency*	*Percentage*
Not aware	8	9.20
PHC – Sub center/MAY	75	86.21
Anganwadi – diet scheme	26	29.89
Immunization	22	25.29
Sanitation	5	5.75
Padha Swayam Sevak	2	2.30
Dai baithak yojana	9	10.34
Health check-up camps	5	5.75
Family Planning	2	2.30

Information Extension regarding the Schemes

Table 8.63

Showing who informed the couples regarding the schemes

Value label	*Frequency*	*Percentage*
Aganwadi sevika	31	35.63
Dai	2	2.30
Doctor	20	22.99
Gramsevak/Member/panchayat	4	4.60
MPW/helper	6	6.90
ANM	73	83.91
Villagers/friends/neighbours	7	8.05
Confused	3	3.45

It would be seen from the data presented that 83.91% of the couples came to know about the schemes from the ANM, this indicates the constant interaction that the villagers have with the ANM. 35.63% came to know about the schemes from Anganwadi sevika; 22.99% came to know about it from the doctors; 8.5% came to know from the villagers, friends and neighbours; 6.9% came to know from the Multi purpose worker and the helper; 4.6% came to know from the gramsevak or the pnchayat members; 2.3 came to know from the dai; and 3.45% were confused about their response.

Opinion about Infrastructural Facilities Related to Health

Table 8.64

Showing opinion about infrastructural facilities related to health, available in the village

Value label	*Frequency*	*Percentage*
Problem during rainy season, non-availability of concerned people	8	9.20
Non-availability of beds	4	4.60
Non-availability of toilet facilities	3	3.45
Facilities available regarding diagnosis and check up	1	1.15
Non-availability of treatment facilities for emergency cases	13	14.94
Poor/inadequate infra structure facilities	34	39.08
Good/adequate facilities	38	43.68
No Response	3	3.45

It would be seen from the data presented that 43.68% of couples said that the facilities available are good and adequate. 39.08% said that the facilities are poor and inadequate; 14.94% couples said that there are no facilities during emergencies; 9.2% couples said that there occur a lot of problems during monsoons and even the concerned doctors and other PHC staff are not available.

It would be seen from the data presented that 85.06% find the schemes useful and 12.64% do not find them useful. 2.3% couples are confused about the response.

Usefulness of Government Schemes

Table 8.65

Showing whether they find the government schemes useful or not

Value label	*Frequency*	*Percentage*
Yes	74	85.06
No	11	12.64
Confused	2	2.30
Grand Total	**87**	**100.00**

Interest in Knowing Government Schemes

Table 8.66

Showing whether they have taken interest in knowing about government schemes and facilities

Value label	*Frequency*	*Percentage*
Yes	63	72.41
No	16	18.39
Confused	8	9.20
Grand Total	**87**	**100.00**

It would be seen from the data presented that 72.41% couples have taken interest in knowing about the government schemes and facilities, 18.39% have not done so and 9.2% are confused about the decision.

Conduciveness of Village Environment

Table 8.67

Showing whether they find the village environment conducive enough to use these facilities

Value label	*Frequency*	*Percentage*
Yes	64	73.56
No	23	26.44
Grand Total	**87**	**100.00**

It would be seen from the data presented that 73.56% couples have expressed positively, whereas 26.44% have expressed negatively.

Benefits of Various Schemes

Table 8.68 a

Showing the schemes they have benefited from

Scheme	*Frequency*	*Percentage*
Food grains given by the government	1	1.15
Matrutva Anudan Yojana	79	90.81
Dai scheme	4	4.60
Diet through anganwadi	19	21.84
Water purification	3	3.45
Medicines provided	4	4.60
Immunization	6	6.90
Prasuti (delivery) benefit scheme	1	1.15
Safe delivery Kit scheme	1	1.15
Health Camps	1	1.15

It would be seen from the data presented that 90.81% couples, that is the majority have benefited from the Matrutva Anudan Yojana; 21.84% have benefited from the diet provided through anganwadis; 6.9 have benefited from immunization for pregnant mothers; 4.6% each have benefited from dai scheme and medicines provided by the PHC; 3.45% couples have benefited from the water purification scheme; and 1.15% each have benefited from food grains provided by the government, benefits during delivery of a child, safe delivery kit scheme and health camps.

It would be seen from the data presented that 69.6% couples have received money along with food and medicines; 68.73% have received only medicine; 30.45% have received only food. 2.61% couples have complained about receiving no help from the ANM at all, whereas 9.57% have received benefits of immunization.

Details of Benefits Received

Table 8.68 b

Showing what benefits the beneficiaries have received

Value label	*Frequency*	*Percentage*
Money	80	69.6
Only food	35	30.45
Only medicine	79	68.73
No benefits from ANM at all	3	2.61
Immunization	11	9.57

Adequacy of Schemes

Table 8.69

Showing whether the beneficiaries find the scheme adequate or not

Value label	*Frequency*	*Percentage*
Yes	69	79.31
No	18	20.69
Grand Total	**87**	**100.00**

It would be seen from the data presented that 79.31% of the couples find the schemes adequate, whereas 20.69% couples find the schemes inadequate.

Hurdles in Getting Benefits of Schemes

Table 8.70

Showing what difficulties the beneficiaries face in getting the scheme

Value label	*Frequency*	*Percentage*
Delay in getting money	26	29.89
All women do not get the benefits of the scheme	2	2.30
There exists partiality in selection of beneficiaries	1	1.15
Nobody provides the information about the scheme	9	10.34
No cooperation	3	3.45
No difficulties	43	49.43
Non availability of stock, irregularity in distribution	4	4.60
Total amount is never paid	6	6.90

It would be seen from the data presented that 58.63% of the couples have expressed about various difficulties like delay in getting money, partiality in selection of beneficiaries, lack of information and cooperation, non availability of stock, irregularity in distribution of benefits and that total amount is never paid. 49.43% couples however said that they do not face any difficulties in getting the scheme.

Approach in Getting Benefit of the Schemes

Table 8.71

Showing whom did the beneficiaries approach in getting the benefit of the scheme

Value label	*Frequency*	*Percentage*
ANM	77	88.51
Multi Purpose Worker	3	3.45
Gram-sewak	3	3.45
Anganwadi sevika	12	13.79
Dai	5	5.75
Doctor	24	27.59
Sarpanch	3	3.45
Talathi	1	1.15
Friend/Neighbour	3	3.45
Confused – no response	3	3.45

It would be seen from the data presented that 88.51% couples approached the ANM for getting the benefits of the schemes; 27.59% couples approached the doctor; 13.79% couples approached the anganwadi sevika; 5.75% couples approached the dai; 3.45% couples each approached Sarpanch, Gramsevak, friends and MPW; and 1.15% couples have approached the talathi in the village.

It would be seen from the data presented that 79.31% couples did not take their difficulties to the higher officials, 4.6% couples felt that it was not needed, and only 16.09 couples really took their difficulties to the higher officials.

Approaching Higher Officials in Case of Difficulty

Table 8.72

Showing whether they took their difficulties to higher officials

Value label	*Frequency*	*Percentage*
Yes	14	16.09
Not needed	4	4.60
No	69	79.31
Grand Total	**87**	**100.00**

Response of the Officials to the Complaints

Table 8.73

Showing the response of the officials after taking the complaints to them

Value label	*Frequency*	*Percentage*
Gave assurance	6	6.90
Not paid attention	8	9.20
Not applicable	73	83.91
Grand Total	**87**	**100.00**

It would be seen from the data presented that 9.2% of the couples responded that the officials did not pay any attention; and 6.9% couples responded that the officials gave assurance of help.

It would be seen from the data presented that 52.87% couples responded that the Medical Officer visits the village once in a week or a fortnight as a part of the flying squad; 28.74% couples responded that the officials visit the village, but not very regularly; whereas 14.94% couples said that the health officials do not visit the village.

Visits of the Higher Officials to the Village

Table 8.74

Showing whether the higher officials like DHO, MO visit their village

Value label	*Frequency*	*Percentage*
MO as a part of flying squad visits once in a week/fortnight	46	52.87
Yes – but irregular visits	25	28.74
No	13	14.94
No response	3	3.45
Grand Total	87	100.00

Satisfaction of Beneficiaries with the Services Provided

Table 8.75

Showing whether the beneficiaries are satisfied with the service provided by the government

Value label	*Frequency*	*Percentage*
Inadequate health facilities – non availability of permanent doctor	25	28.74
Disturbance and interference – problems due to tiger project	30	34.48
Non–availability of nurse and MPW	1	1.15
Irregularity of health officials	9	10.34
Lack of services in emergency cases	3	3.45
Partiality in distributions of schemes	18	20.69
Satisfied	23	26.44
Delay in services and scheme benefits	6	6.90

It would be seen from the data presented that 34.48% couples expressed that they are facing a lot of disturbance and interference due to the implementation of the Tiger project in the area. 28.74% couples expressed regarding inadequate health facilities and non-availability of the permanent doctors; 20.69% couples have expressed unhappiness regarding the partiality in distribution of schemes; 10.34% couples have spoken about irregularity of health officials;

6.9% have expressed regarding the delay in services and scheme benefits; 3.45% couples have expressed regarding the lack of services in emergency cases. 26.44% couples have expressed satisfaction regarding the services provided by the government.

Employees of Primary Health Center

A set of questions were asked to the employees/staff of the Primary Health Center of Semadoh, Chikhaldara block as all the beneficiaries interviewed are from the villages falling under the purview of Semadoh PHC.

The following tables focus on: The training received by the staff; Their work profile; Their knowledge regarding government schemes; Their role in implementation of government schemes; Their opinion about the adequacy of infrastructural facilities in the village; Their suggestions for improvement of these facilities; The adequacy of attention being given to the health factor; The relevance and adequacy of government policies and schemes related to health; The knowledge of specific schemes related to reproductive health of women; The problems faced in disseminating information about these schemes; The critical aspects of the problems faced by people related to government schemes; The social problems faced while doing work related to schemes; The reasons for low awareness of people about the government facilities and schemes; and the government measures to improve facilities and quality of services.

It would be seen from the data presented that 33.33% of the staff falls into the age-group of 25-30 years; 33.33 fall into the age-group of 30-35 years; and the remaining 33.33% fall into the higher age-group of 40-55 years.

Age-wise Status of the Employees

Table 8.76

Showing age of the employees

Value Label – age	*Frequency*	*Percentage*
28	1	6.67
29	2	13.33
30	2	13.33
32	3	20.00
33	1	6.67
35	1	6.67
41	1	6.67
42	2	13.33
46	1	6.67
53	1	6.67
Grand Total	**15**	**100.00**

Sex-wise Distribution of the Employees

Table 8.77

Showing sex distribution of the employees

Value Label	*Frequency*	*Percentage*
F	6	40.00
M	9	60.00
Grand Total	**15**	**100.00**

It would be seen from the data presented that 60% of the staff members are males and 40% of the staff members are females.

The caste wise, religion wise and education wise distribution of the employees is as follows:

Caste-wise Distribution of Employees

Table 8.78

Caste wise distribution of the employees

Value Label	*Frequency*	*Percentage*
Balai	1	6.67
Brahman	1	6.67
Buddhist	2	13.33
Christian	1	6.67
Costi	1	6.67
Dhangar	1	6.67
Korku	3	20.00
Kunbi	2	13.33
Mali	1	6.67
Nhavi	2	13.33
Grand Total	**15**	**100.00**

Religion-wise Distribution of Employees

Table 8.79

Religion wise distribution of the employees

Value Label	*Frequency*	*Percentage*
Christian	1	6.67
Hindu	14	93.33
Grand Total	**15**	**100.00**

Education-wise Distribution of Employees

Table 8.80

Education wise distribution of the employees

Value Label	*Frequency*	*Percentage*
Illiterate	1	6.67
7th std	1	6.67
S.S.C.	3	20.00
11 th std	2	13.33
H.S.C.	4	26.67
B.A.M.S.	3	20.00
M.B.B.S.	1	6.67
Grand Total	**15**	**100.00**

Trainings Received by the Staff

Table 8.81

Showing the trainings received by the staff members

Value Label	*Frequency*	*Percentage*
HMIS	4	26.67
Training in Reproductive and Child Health	12	80.00
Training in Malaria prevention	1	6.67
Tuberculosis and Leprosy training	11	73.33
Training in nutrition and gradation	1	6.67
Operating safe delivery kits	1	6.67
Training in sanitation	1	6.67
Training in MCH and CSSM	2	13.33
Special training for the handicapped	1	6.67
Diploma in Health Education	4	26.67
Family Planning and AIDS	1	6.67

It would be seen from the data presented that 80% of the staff members have received training in RCH; 73.33% have received training in tuberculosis and leprosy cure; 26.67% have received training in HMIS; 26.67 have completed a one year diploma course in health education. Several other types of training have been received by the staff members like malaria prevention, nutrition and gradation, operating of safe delivery kits, sanitation, for the handicapped and MCH and CSSM.

Work Profile of the Staff Members

Table 8.82

Showing the work profile of the staff members

Value Label	*Frequency*	*Percentage*
Treatment and testing/grading/supply	6	40.00
Awareness creation and information dissemination	4	26.67
Supervision of grass-root level workers.	11	73.33
Extension of schemes and selection of beneficiaries	9	60.00
OPD	5	33.33
Cross-checking the beneficiaries	2	13.33
Field visits/home visits	6	40.00
Linkages with other line departments	1	6.67

It would be seen from the data presented that 73.33% staff members are involved in supervision of grass root level workers; 60% in selection of beneficiaries and extension of schemes; 40% staff has to pay home and field visits; 40% are involved in treatment, testing, grading and supply activities; 33.33% are involved in the OPD activities; 13.33% staff cross-checks the benefits received by the beneficiaries; 6.67% are responsible for establishing linkages with the line departments; and only 26.67% of the staff is responsible for awareness creation and information dissemination work.

It would be seen from the data presented that more than 60% of the staff members are knowledgeable about Dai training scheme, Flying Squad scheme and Matrutva Anudan Yojana; between 20 and 50% staff members are knowledgeable about Padha swayam sevak scheme, RCH program, schemes for malnourished children, ICDS scheme, Nucleus Budget scheme and Family Planning Scheme. Very few staff members have spoken about Prasuti Arthsahayya Yojana, immunization, water purification and Nav-Sanjivani scheme. It is rather surprising that a scheme as important as Nav-Sanjivani has been mentioned, only by one staff member.

Knowledge regarding Government Schemes

Table 8.83

Showing the knowledge regarding government schemes

Value Label	*Frequency*	*Percentage*
Dai training scheme	9	60.00
Padha Swayam Sevak scheme	7	46.67
Flying squad	9	60.00
MAY	10	66.67
RCH program	5	33.33
Malnourished children scheme	4	26.67
ICDS scheme	3	20.00
Nucleus budget scheme	4	26.67
Prasuti Arthasahayya yojana	1	6.67
Family Planning scheme	5	33.33
Immunization	1	6.67
Water purification scheme	1	6.67
Nav-sanjivani Yojana	1	6.67

It would be seen from the data presented that 73.33% of staff members are involved in awareness generation work; 33.3% undertake follow up of the schemes with the beneficiaries and cross check with them; more than 40% staff members undertake supervision and implementation of RCH program; 40% do the registration and selection of the beneficiaries; and 20% are involved in distribution of money and medicine as well as undertaking individual and group meetings.

Role of the Staff Members

Table 8.84

Showing the role of the staff members in implementation of government schemes

Value Label	*Frequency*	*Percentage*
Awareness generation and info dissemination	11	73.33
Follow-up of the scheme with the beneficiaries	5	33.33
Cross check the beneficiaries	5	33.33
Supervise, guide and help grass root level workers	7	46.67
Implementing RCH activities	6	40.00
Distribution of money and medicine	3	20.00
Reporting to MO	4	26.67
Registration and selection of beneficiaries	6	40.00
Individual and group meetings	3	20.00

Opinions of Staff Members regarding Adequacy of Infrastructural Facilities

Table 8.85 a

Showing the opinions of the staff members regarding the adequacy of infrastructural facility in the village

Value Label	*Frequency*	*Percentage*
Adequate	5	33.33
Problem related to warm room	4	26.67
Separate delivery room village wise is needed	6	40.00
Non availability of space	2	13.33
Poor communication facilities	1	6.67
Quarters for MPW required	3	20.00
Regular repairs and maintenance required	5	33.33

It would be seen from the data presented that 40% of the staff feels the need of separate delivery room in every village. 33.3% staff feels that the facilities are adequate; 33.3% feels that regular repairs and maintenance is required; 26.67% fell that there are problems related to the warm rooms that have been established recently as a part of Melghat pattern; 20% staff has spoken about the requirement of quarters for the MPWs; 13.33% said about non-availability of space; and 6.67% have expressed regarding poor communication facilities.

Suggestions of the Staff Members regarding Improvements

Table 8.85 b

Showing the suggestions of the staff members regarding improvement of these facilities

Value Label	*Frequency*	*Percentage*
None	1	6.67
Yearly/annual maintenance	6	40.00
Telephone and electric facilities	1	6.67
Construction of separate delivery room	4	26.67
Flying squad should be throughout the year	2	13.33
Permanent staff at sub-center	2	13.33
Village wise dispensary and child-care unit	6	40.00
Quarters for MPW and the stock supply in time	2	13.33

It would be seen from the data presented that 40% of the staff has suggested that regular and annual maintenance work should be undertaken as well as village wise dispensary and child care units should be established; 26.67% staff members suggested that construction of a separate delivery room should be done; 13.33% suggested that the flying squad machinery should be working throughout the year, there should be a permanent staff at the sub-center, quarters should be provided to MPW, and the stock supply should be done in time. 6.67% staff has suggested to improve the telephone and electric facilities.

Adequacy of Attention to Health Factor

Table 8.86

Showing whether adequate attention is being given to the health factor

Value Label	*Frequency*	*Percentage*
Lack of sanitation and hygiene	3	20.00
Special schemes for Melghat	1	6.67
Adequate attention	14	93.33
Illiteracy should be reduced	1	6.67
Visits of doctors as per people's convenience	1	6.67

It would be seen from the data presented that 93.3% have expressed that adequate attention is being paid to the health factor in the Melghat region. However, 20% of staff has also expressed that there exist lack of sanitation and hygiene facilities; 6.67% have felt that there should be more special schemes for Melghat, illiteracy should be reduced and visits of the doctors should be arranged as per the convenience of people.

Relevance and Adequacy of Government Policies

Table 8.87

Showing whether the government policies regarding health are relevant and adequate

Value Label	*Frequency*	*Percentage*
Yes	6	40.00
No	7	46.67
Confused	2	13.33
Grand Total	**15**	**100.00**

It would be seen from the data presented that 46.67% staff feels that the government policies are not relevant and adequate; 40% feel that they are adequate enough and 13.33% are confused.

Relevance and Adequacy of Health Schemes

Table 8.88

Showing whether the government schemes related to health relevant and adequate

Value Label	*Frequency*	*Percentage*
Yes	5	33.33
No	10	66.67
Grand Total	**15**	**100.00**

It would be seen from the data presented that 66.67% have responded negatively and 33.3% have responded positively.

Specific Schemes related to Reproductive Health of Women

Table 8.89

Showing whether there any specific schemes related to reproductive health of women

Value Label	*Frequency*	*Percentage*
Matrutva Anudan Yojana	14	93.33
ICDS /anganwadi scheme	7	46.67
Pantpradhan Jawahar Yojana – nutrition for women	1	6.67
Nucleus Budget Scheme	6	40.00
Dai Baithak Yojana	5	33.33
Scheme for malnourished child	10	66.67
Family Planning Scheme	1	6.67
Immunization for the pregnant and newborn child	2	13.33

It would be seen from the data presented that 93.33% staff members have mentioned about the Matrutva Anudan Yojana; 66.67% have spoken about food availability for malnourished children; 46.67% have mentioned regarding the availability of diet for pregnant and nursing mothers through the Anganwadis, under the ICDS program; 40% have mentioned the Nucleus Budget scheme being provided by the Integrated Tribal Development Project, Dharni;

33.33% have mentioned the Dai training scheme. Apart from this the staff has also mentioned about the Pantpradahan Jawahar Yojana, which provides with nutrition for women, the Family Planning scheme implemented by PHCs, and the immunization program both for the children and mothers.

Possibility of Problems in Information Dissemination

Table 8.90

Showing whether the employees face any problem in disseminating information about these schemes

Value Label	*Frequency*	*Percentage*
Yes	10	66.67
No	5	33.33
Grand Total	**15**	**100.00**

It would be seen from the data presented that 66.7% of the staff faces problems in disseminating information about the schemes, whereas 33.3% feels that they do not face any such problem in doing so.

Problems Faced in Information Dissemination

Table 8.91

Showing the problems faced by the staff in disseminating information about these schemes

Value Label	*Frequency*	*Percentage*
Language problem – do not know Korku language	6	40.00
Low level of understanding amongst Korkus due to illiteracy	4	26.67
Beneficiaries complain about partiality and do not respond well	1	6.67
Non availability of beneficiaries due to farming and Mahua season	1	6.67
Pressures from village leaders	1	6.67
Pressures from Gavali community for benefits	1	6.67
Disunity of villagers and groupism	1	6.67
N.A.	5	33.33

It would be seen from the data presented that 40% of the staff members have identified language problem, that is not knowing the Korku language for communication, as one of the major problems faced by them. 26.67% have mentioned that due to prevalence of illiteracy, the Korkus are not able to understand many things while disseminating information. Other problems quoted by the staff are: poor response of beneficiaries due to complain about partiality in distribution of schemes and benefits; non availability of beneficiaries due to farming and Mahua season; pressures from village leaders; and pressures from Gavali community for benefits. 33.33% of the staff members have refrained from mentioning the problems.

Criticality of Problems Faced related to Government Schemes

Table 8.92

Showing whether the problems faced by people related to these government schemes are critical

Value Label	*Frequency*	*Percentage*
No	14	93.33
Yes	1	6.67
Grand Total	**15**	**100.00**

It would be seen from the data presented that 93.3% have responded that there exist no such critical problems, whereas 6.67% feel that problems faced by people related to these government schemes are critical.

It would be seen from the data presented that 46.67% staff members have identified the pressures of political leaders as one of the major social problem. 26.67% of the staff has mentioned regarding internal problems and groupism in the village, belief of Korkus in Bhagats and Bhumkas and distrust in PHC treatment as social problems. One staff member has specifically talked about the opposition from other communities in the area, mainly because the special schemes are meant for the tribals, that is Korkus and Gonds. 13.33% feels that they do not encounter and social problems while doing their work.

Extent of Social Problems Faced by the Staff

Table 8.93

Showing what social problems the staff faces while doing the work related to schemes

Value Label	*Frequency*	*Percentage*
No problems	2	13.33
Internal problems and groupism in village	4	26.67
Belief in Bhagat and Bhumka	4	26.67
Distrust in PHC treatment	4	26.67
Pressures of Political leadership amongst the village	7	46.67
Preference to home based treatment and delivery	1	6.67
RCH only for Korku and Gond – hence opposition from others	1	6.67

Reasons for Low Awareness of People

Table 8.94

Showing what are the reasons according to the staff for low awareness of people regarding the government facilities and schemes

Value Label	*Frequency*	*Percentage*
Unemployment and low income	14	93.33
Illiteracy and low level of understanding	12	80.00
Unprotected farming	12	80.00
Inefficient PHC staff	2	13.33
Transport and communication problems	2	13.33
Disinterest amongst villagers	3	20.00
Belief in Bhagat, Bhumka, Padiyal	1	6.67
Language problem	1	6.67

It would be seen from the data presented that 93.33%, majority of the staff members have spoken about unemployment and low income as the most critical problems of the tribal people in the area, leading to their disinterest in most of the things around. 80% mentioned regarding the prevalence of illiteracy and unprotected farming as the reason for low awareness, as the people are engaged and busy in protecting their farms from the wild animals, whom they cannot kill due to forest laws, even if they destroy the farms. Transport and communication problems as well as inefficiency of PHC staff has been mentioned as reasons for low awareness. Apart from this, the belief of Korkus in the traditional healers and the language problem is cited as reasons for low awareness.

Government Measures Undertaken to Improve Facilities & Services

Table 8.95

Showing what government measures have been taken to improve these facilities and quality of services

Value Label	*Frequency*	*Percentage*
Educational facilities	10	66.67
Employment through EGS	4	26.67
PHC facility and flying squad	10	66.67
Adult education	1	6.67
Anganwadis	3	20.00
Ashram schools	4	26.67
Road development	4	26.67
IEC programs	2	13.33
Yearly food for BPL	1	6.67
Huts and construction	2	13.33

It would be seen from the data presented that 66.67% of staff members spoke about provision of educational facilities and public health facilities along with the flying squad to inspect the machinery from time to time. 26.67% of the staff members have spoken about the Employment Guarantee Scheme, the ashram schools for the tribal children, and the road development taken place in last ten years. 20% have accredited the work of anganwadis; and 13.33% have spoken about IEC programs and huts provided by the government. 6.67% have spoken about the adult education program and the yearly food provided to the families falling Below Poverty Line.

9

Conclusions and Recommendations

The present chapter presents the conclusions of the impact analysis study and further lays down the following recommendations.

Conclusions and Recommendations

1. Contents of the National and State Health Policies

As highlighted in the entire study, the content of the policies both at the central and state level reflect an excellent quality of content in terms of the designing of programs, the needs assessment undertaken at all levels, the expertise utilized in doing so, and the efficacy of entire policy making process. The study has identified the gaps between the actual policy making and policy implementation process and hence, it is important to note that though the policies seem adequate enough, the implementation mechanisms leave much to be desired and therefore the need for more effective and efficient implementation strategies are required.

2. Reproductive Health Policies and Programs

All the policy documents since independence have talked about women's health in the context of Population Control and Family Planning. The initial women oriented health programs like 'Maternal and Child Health' as the name rightly reflects focused mainly upon the immunization and prenatal and postnatal requirements, though important enough at a time when India had to ensure that at least all the mothers are getting immunized and are following the procedures for delivering a healthy child. Till almost five decades, the focus remained the same, until the ICPD, Cairo forced the country to revise and shift its focus.

Though the country has launched the Reproductive and Child Health programs in almost all the parts, one does not come across a National Reproductive Health Policy of India, like the National Health or National Population Policy. However, it is interesting as well as ironical to note that the entire National Population Policy 2000, has such unlimited repetition of the terminology – Reproductive and Child Health, that it would not be wrong for a reader to mistake it as National RCH Policy, if he/she is furnished with the document without the cover page.

Though a number of officials at the implementation level have stated that there is no difference in the present RCH program than the earlier ones, it is high time that the policy makers percolate the need to understand the difference with regards to the present program and the new approach amongst the policy implementers. There definitely arises the need to understand the shift in the approach and avoid the target oriented, time bound approach and style of functioning.

The initial policy statements were mainly incorporated in the National and State Family Planning Program, further a more detailed outlay of the policies emerged in the National Health Policy – 1983 and subsequently in the State Health Policies. Today, a lot of reproductive health aspects are looked at in the National as well as State Population Policies. It would be more appropriate that the country as well as state has a complete and comprehensive health policy, covering and catering to all the health programs and also ensuring its inter linkages. For example, the RTI/STI education programs, though a part of the RCH program in the country and the states, is being carried out by the State AIDS Control Societies, this definitely needs to be stated and interlinked at the policy level, which will in turn ensure easy and clear implementation of the same. There has to be total integration in all the wings, that is the Ministry of Health, Family Welfare, National AIDS Control Organization (NACO), all the state Ministries and all the special area projects.

3. Necessity to Shift Focus from Quantitative to Qualitative Aspects

The Family Welfare wing of the Public Health Department has done remarkable work in last 55 years with regard to the quantitative aspects, but it has lagged behind in providing qualitative reproductive health services as well as even in terms of raising the confidence of both men and women in undertaking an informed choice, as the entire Family Planning (till 1976) and Family Welfare (after 1976) program has been lopsided and has concentrated upon female sterilization. The quantitative growths can be measured by the increase infrastructural facilities and the raising of number of clinics meant for exclusively Family Welfare activities. The number of PHCs and Sub-centers has gone up remarkably.

And, like any other usual developmental program in the country, as a result of the quantitative growth in Primary Health and because of the preoccupation with the goals like Health For All; the need for looking at the qualitative aspect took a back seat. Besides, the needs and more important the poverty of the rural and tribal people has not been given due consideration. Poverty, inaccessibility and lack of knowledge is the worst hindrance to the safety and reproductive health care of adolescents and women. Without eliminating poverty and meeting the basic minimum needs like food, water, roads, electricity, public transport, education, and the means of livelihood for a burgeoning population the cause for quality health care in general and reproductive health care in particular cannot be advanced.

4. Implementation Mechanisms of Health Policies

As explained by most of the officials, the implementation process is extremely smooth, but at the same time it is equally true that a lot of pressure has been exerted by the state government in cases where some kind of crisis has taken place in past few years. It is important to note that extra efforts in a crisis struck Amravati district have resulted in a complete set of schemes called Melghat Pattern, at the same time it should also be noted that similar schemes have yet to be replicated and implemented in other districts of Maharashtra. Several governments have witnessed till date that unless there are pressures, crises or emergency situations the efficacy of implementation mechanisms cannot be detected.

5. Decade-wise Changes in the MCH Programs and the Final Designing of RCH

A complete merger of all the erstwhile programs into the RCH program in India has resulted into implementation of a number of programs under the banner of RCH. However, today also the so called RCH program is not acutely focusing upon the day to day reproductive health problems faced by the women in either the rural or tribal areas. Most of the women interviewed responded that they are told about family planning, sanitation and hygiene and general health care, but still do not have a clue regarding their regular problems like white discharge, abdominal pains, or even vaginal irritation, not only is it difficult to tackle but at the same time it is not possible to discuss it with anybody and the accessibility of the doctor or any other medical staff is still felt as a remote possibility. Apart from this there are problems related to reproductive tract like the reproductive tract and cervical cancers, which are not prioritized by the Public Health due to lack of treatment facilities as well as the cost. Despite all the efforts in the various programs like MCH, CSSM and the present RCH, most women in the rural areas still have non institutional deliveries, do not register themselves even after the completion of two trimesters and do not take the immunization.

The World Bank team assembled in India in 1994 to help the Indian Government "carry out the commitment given at the Cairo population conference to implement a client-centered approach" to Reproductive Health and Family Planning services. A proposed package of essential Reproductive and Child Health services for the Public Health system, with focus on reproductive tract and sexually transmitted infections in India was drawn upon. And a review of Family Welfare Program's management information and evaluation system was undertaken. The World Bank team can be credited with the achievement of convincing the Indian government to reconsider the merits of its target system. In 1995, the government agreed to remove targets from two districts in the state of Uttar Pradesh so that the viability of a target-free program could be studied. Simultaneously, it withdrew targets from one district in every state of the country and gradually one year later, the government declared the entire country target-free[1]. Though the government calls the whole approach as target free, the achievements of each district are still calculated in terms of physical works undertaken rather than the calculation of outreach with regards to information extended and problems tackled of a particular number of families.

6. Financial Sustainability of Programs

The financial sustainability of all the programs being implemented presently always remains a question to be answered, as the Public Health System in India does not have sources that ensure cost recovery. The nominal fee of Rs. 2 at the PHC really does not bring in any income to the department. In the years to come the Central as well as State governments will have to ensure the financial provisions rather than remain dependent on donors.

Very recently, the Central Government has stopped the financial assistance being extended to all the Post Partum Centers being managed by the Governmental Agencies, Non-governmental Organizations and Municipal Corporations. There has been a general hue and cry over this sudden decision and hence, all the concerned agencies have been demanding these ongoing funds which, they have been receiving for last 4-5 decades. Though financial exigencies have compelled the Central Government to take this decision, it has also looked into the actual performance of these centers. With the well established and growing private health care services, it has not only reduced the clientele visiting these centers, but at the same time, there hardly is any enthusiasm amongst the staff of these centers.

7. Political Stability

Political stability of the system has a positive impact on the continuity in the implementation of the programs. Frequent changes both, at the Ministerial level and the Bureaucratic level create hindrances in this process of implementation.

8. Panchayati Raj Institutions and Reproductive Health Care

The elected female representatives of the Gram Panchayats need to play a more active role in promoting awareness about reproductive health of women and their independence by representing their interests in the developmental activities of the Gram Panchayat. The Panchayati Raj representatives are in a continuous contact with the Panchayat Samitee at the block level and get all the information regarding the schemes, which they can use for implementing health programs for women. One can argue in favour of conducting workshops at the Gram Panchayat level for these representatives to generate awareness about the approach to be taken to secure the facilities.

9. Adequacy of Schemes for Reproductive Health Care

The local village communities have become more vigilant about the provision of health facilities and several health schemes being extended by the state and central government. A number of couples complained about the incidences of failures of tubectomies and the irritation thereafter; the failure of vasectomies and the break-ups in several families and harassment of women due to it; the problems faced by women in emergency problems like still births and difficult pregnancies and the lack of emergency facilities in such instances; the natural and unnatural abortions occurring in women and the dangers arising from lack of health care in such situations. Apart from the non-availability of facilities during emergencies, a number of couples benefiting from the schemes talked about frauds and delays in actual procurement of benefits. Most of the time the administrative procedures have resulted into such long delays that the purpose of the benefits extended has been defeated.

The officials from the Directorate of Health Services, Mumbai, have also accepted the failures regarding disbursement of benefits due to administrative procedures. It is recommended that for a smooth extension of these schemes two arrangements are extremely necessary: One – the financial disbursement should be done directly and immediately through the Public Health Department rather than the procedure of distribution through the BDOs office at block level. Two – the renewal of schemes should be made every five years rather than every year, so that the delay in renewals every year causing the further delay in disbursement of benefits shall be avoided.

10. Requirement of Qualitative Training and the Role of the IEC

Extension of qualitative training to the health personnel involved in IEC is crucial for the qualitative improvement of reproductive health care. Training would equip the health personnel with the skills for inculcating a sense of understanding, confidence and information/awareness amongst the women. The information from the State IEC Bureau reveals that there are hardly any DEMOs or other personnel of the IEC units at district level who are technically and formally qualified enough for their jobs. This lacuna may be rectified by effective training of the available personnel.

11. Need of Special Grants for Local Initiatives in IEC

With the burgeoning Panchayati Raj Institutions at the block and village level, it would be more appropriate to provide with special grants for local initiatives in IEC program.

12. Requirement of Man-power in IEC Units

The inadequacy of the staff at the district level IEC units has raised a lot of questions: Firstly, the non-availability of the qualified officials suitable for the position of District Education Media Officers (DEMOs). Due to the non-recruitment in the government several positions are not being filled up after a lapse of vacancy of a period of six months. The position of a DEMO is a Class II position under the Maharashtra government to be filled in through the Maharashtra Public Service Commission (MPSC) examinations. This recruitment has also been stalled since several years. As an alternative the government has filled positions of DEMOs in the entire state with deputed officials of Class III grade. It is also interesting to note that even for deputation to this position one has to possess a post graduate degree, should have completed a one year diploma course of Diploma in Health Education provided by the Public health Department and should be in a position of Health Assistant. This qualification is not possessed by most of the deputed officers. Secondly, the other positions at the IEC units are also not filled up so that the unit can function successfully. Hence it is necessary that the state looks into the filling up of these positions and treat the IEC units with equal importance in the entire health structure.

It is also important to note the other common cause of non-availability of officials at block and village level and the non-willingness of the qualified officials to work at these levels. The reasons given by the officials for this are lack of education and communication facilities, unwillingness of the family members to shit to the local areas and so on.

13. Differences Between Medical and Non-medical Officials

The officials from both the Directorate of Health Services and the State IEC Bureau argued that a number of times a program like IEC suffers due to the differences of opinion between the medical and non-medical personnel in the Public Health Department. The medical personnel feel that they are best qualified to decide what is to be communicated and how, whereas the non-medical personnel feel that it is them who can really design and define the strategies for IEC. Though this gap/chasm between the two is not new, as even the State Minister for Health accepted this rigidity amongst both the groups, but with growing applicability and requirement of IEC this needs to be overcome and appropriately balanced.

14. Emphasis on Male Participation and NSV

India has defined a basic package of essential RCH services based on the requirements of ICPD, finally eliminating the method-specific targets, which is especially important for female sterilization procedures. The pre-1996 period focused upon essentially one-method program of female sterilization as the predominant means of contraception, leaving no choice for women. These services too were mostly provided in camps that lacked time or equipment for proper infection prevention measures as well as time to counsel clients, with hardly any efforts of follow-up in the cases of complications. Promotion of male methods was hardly undertaken after the Family Planning Drive in the seventies and the subsequent fall of the then ruling government. No government after that has ever risked itself in undertaking such drives, however the present efforts in promotion of NSV need to be seriously planned in the rural areas, as the concept, the benefits as well as the simplicity of this so called operation is not very much known to men in rural areas and they still visualize the earlier system and procedures of vasectomies.

15. Sensitization and Not Just Skill Based Training

The functioning style of the health personnel at the peripheral level indicates that the message of health conditions and problems faced by the locals has not yet reached to them completely. Though they are very well equipped in terms of professional and specialized skills required to deliver their jobs, they lack the interpersonal skills and sensitivity to the health issues erupting at village level, hence, there is tremendous need to sensitize the health personnel so that they would be able to tackle the problems and emergencies not just through professional skills but with a humane approach.

16. Requirement of Defined Mechanisms for Information Dissemination

The material prepared by the State IEC Bureau is well developed and is capable of extending health education to the people, provided the material is disseminated properly and reaches the right areas where it is required. For example, the publicity boards are used as rooftop material by the locals.

17. IEC Material to Emphasize on Socio-cultural & Local Aspects

IEC material prepared by the state government has to focus upon the socio-cultural and local aspects of the area where the material has to be displayed and disseminated. Unless the audience understands and identifies themselves with the media used for extending and conveying the message, the purpose of the IEC material is defeated. India being a country of varying languages, dialects and cultures it is extremely important that area specific material is produced keeping in mind the specific area based issues. For example the material prepared in Marathi Language is unable to convey the message to the border area audience who belong to Hindi speaking groups like those in the Melghat area.

18. Emphasis to be on Electrical and Electronic Media

Presently the IEC material produced is mostly in print form, due to the constraints of non- availability of electricity or electronic gadgets in the rural areas. However, in an era, where the electronic media has proven its effectiveness in many fields, it is extremely important that more and more IEC material should be produced in electronic form. Though posters and written material has its own impact, electronic media has a faster and long lasting impact, as it comprises of moving pictures and dialogues. A model needs to be established wherein each PHC and Sub-Center should be well equipped with television sets and should display material electronically as is done in public places like railway stations. Apart from this, IEC material through electronic media should be extended in all the hospitals, schools and public places, this will definitely lead to health education through hammering and continuous efforts.

19. Requirement of Coordination and Integration of Efforts

It is self evident, that there will have to be a convergence of all the schemes and programs of the Central Government, State Government and the Panchayati Raj Institutions, as well as coordination of various concerned and associated departments in the social sectors for even one sector like, health to achieve the goal of quality health care.

The Reproductive Health Program has been designed and sponsored by the Central Government, which is further implemented by the State Governments. The Ministry of Health and Family Welfare collaborates with the Ministry of Information and Broadcasting, Ministry of Human Resource Development, the associated departments like Department of Women and Child Development, Department of Education, Ministry of Rural Development, work with a multi-sectoral committee of secretaries from these ministries. A similar structure is required and needs to be worked out at the state level also. Conscious efforts and strategies through such multi-sectoral committees need to be designed and applied in preparing as well as conveying area based and need based messages resulting into health education.

20. Inspection Machinery

Several mechanisms for inspection have been laid down in the earlier chapters. Integrated inspection machinery is required and the following model reflects the involvement of officials at district, division and directorate level.

21. Requirement of Implementation Machinery for Emergency Obstetric Care

Emergency obstetric care is one of the most essential services in the extension of reproductive health care; a number of couples expressed the need for emergency care and the problems arising due to its unavailability. Though, innovative efforts are being made at local level as the ones stated by the DHO Amravati, a standard and uniform machinery is required to be set up at village level, all over India to tackle the issues of emergency obstetric. Unless, a significant aspect like obstetric care is ensured, it would be ironical to declare that the reproductive health services are being extended effectively.

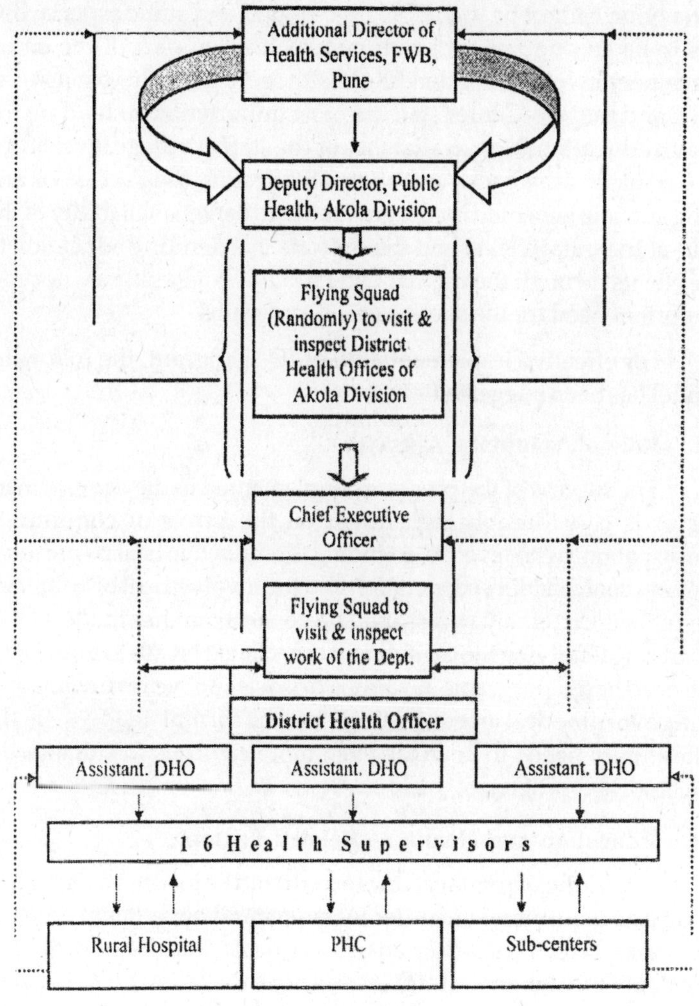

Diagram No. 9.1

22. IEC and Availability of PHC Staff

IEC should not be looked at into the narrow framework of display and dissemination of material and information, but has to be visualized in a broader context. This visualization demands that IEC being an ongoing process aiming at changes in attitude and behaviour, cannot be limited to time-bound and static aspects. IEC has to be an ongoing and continuous effort on part of the entire machinery involved in extending health services. In this context, the PHC and the Sub-Center staff are most important in extending the health education. Non availability of the staff at village level is one of the major drawbacks and shortfall affecting the success of any program implemented by the government, hence, availability of the staff at the village level and their efforts in extending education to the clients through the regular OPD should be assessed as the most important need for the success of IEC programs.

For effective implementation of IEC program, the following model has been suggested

23. Role of Voluntary Agencies

The success of the programs implemented in the development sector is considerably dependent on the levels of community participation, hence even in extending reproductive health care inter-sectoral coordination, cooperation and the involvement of voluntary agencies is extremely necessary. The government has made a lot of efforts in identifying the capable and capacitated NGOs to implement the need based programs in various districts. Active involvement of nongovernmental organizations and informal leaders in the community needs to be made even more rigorous to enhance the effects of IEC programs.

24. Education and Health as Related Factors

Acquiring of primary education should be focused as an urgent and basic requirement in order to understand oneself and enhance personal care. Education ensures a basic understanding and capability to think and act. This aspect is very necessary if the women are to take care of their own reproductive health and are to develop coping mechanisms.

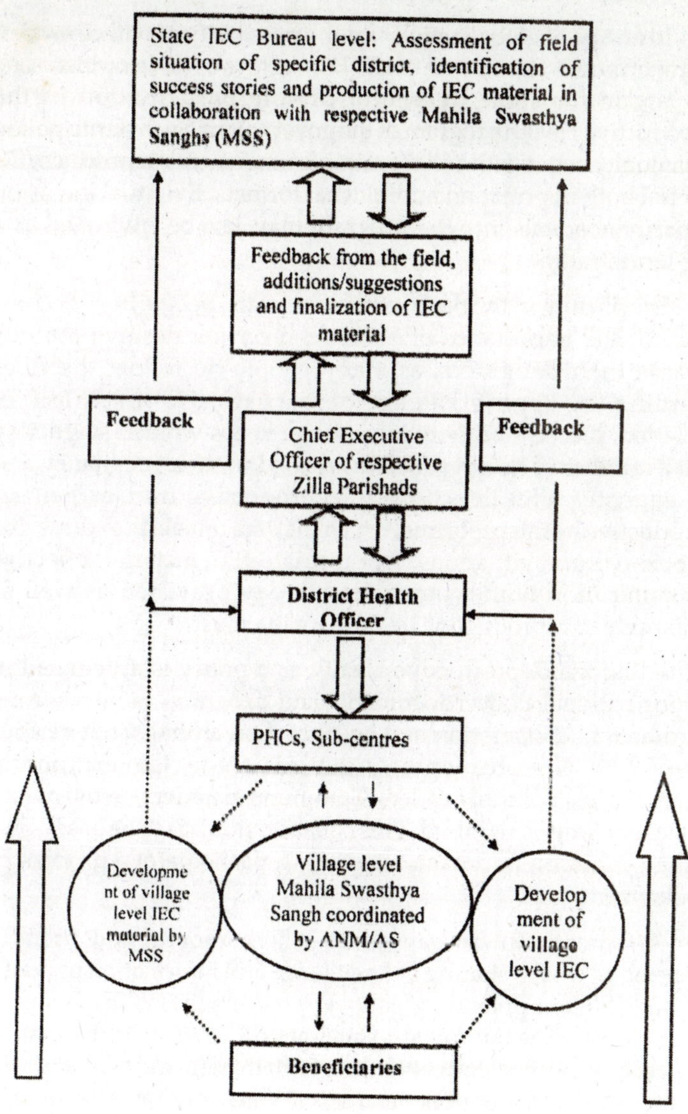

Diagram No. 9.2

Impact Assessment of IEC Material

25. Private Sector Participation

In an age of globalization and the possibility of withdrawal of the government from some of the key sectors of development one may argue for some degree of private participation in the Reproductive Health program of the government. Such participation may initially begin with collaborative arrangements to produce IEC material both in print and audiovisual formats. Eventual inclusion of charity hospitals into the program may also be envisaged as a long-term strategy.

Specifically, in the past twenty-five years, people have become aware of the importance of health and have a positive attitude towards their daughters, as many people do follow the rules regarding the appropriate age of marriage. However, lack of education, inaccessibility to knowledge keeps women stagnating with a number of health problems related to their pregnancy and subsequently with infections in reproductive tract or general reproductive health problems, which they are unable to express due to socio-cultural situations. Appropriate IEC material, effective communication with women, day-to-day provision as well as availability of reproductive health care is a must.

Although Reproductive Health as a policy is articulated in various national policy documents and programs, a very strong coordination, cooperation and collaboration amongst the various actors like Governmental Agencies, Non Governmental Organizations, Political Leaders, Community Leaders, Activists and the stakeholders is required. This collaboration has to be based on a woman-centered approach ensuring a participatory process of development.

A woman-centered approach where a joyful and friendly extension as well as sharing of knowledge and information prevails, will build all four pillars of Quality Reproductive Health of women of our country. The four pillars, Qualitative Knowledge; Qualitative Service; Qualitative Understanding of both men and women; and Qualitative Interactions between service providers and the people are required to be established rather than the bureaucratic and target oriented approach of conducting a particular number of surgeries/ operations; distribution of pills and condoms; and dissemination of a particular quantity of IEC material.

REFERENCES

1. Khan, M.E. and George Cernada (eds.). Spacing as an Alternative Strategy: India's Family Welfare Program (New Delhi: B.R. Publishing Corporation, 1996).

Bibliography

Primary Sources

Annual Report, (Office of Registrar General, India and Ministry of Health and Family Welfare, New Delhi, 2002).

Government of India, *National Population Policy 2000,* (New Delhi, Department of Family Welfare, Government of India, 2000).

Government of India, *Manual on Community Needs Assessment Approach in Family Welfare Program,* (New Delhi, Ministry of Health and Family Welfare, Government of India, 1998).

Government of India, *Reproductive and Child Health Program,* (New Delhi, Ministry of Health and Family Welfare, Government of India, 1997).

1991 Census, Amaravati District, Maharashtra, 1991.

Government of India, Planning Commission, *Document 16,* (New Delhi, 1951).

Government of India, *Towards Equality,* (Report of the Committee on the Status of Women in India, New Delhi, 1974).

Government of India, *Report of Independent Commission on Health in India,* (New Delhi, 1984).

Government of India, *National Health Policy 1983,* (New Delhi, Department of Family Welfare, Govt. of India, 1983).

Government of India, *First Five Year Plan,* (New Delhi, Planning Commission, 1951).

Government of India, *Second Five Year Plan,* (New Delhi, Planning Commission, 1956).

Government of India, *Third Five Year Plan,* (New Delhi, Planning Commission, 1961).

Government of India, *Fourth Five Year Plan,* (New Delhi, Planning Commission, 1966).

Government of India, *Fifth Five Year Plan,* (New Delhi, Planning Commission, 1974).

Government of India, *Sixth Five Year Plan,* (New Delhi, Planning Commission, 1980).

Government of India, *Seventh Five Year Plan,* (New Delhi, Planning Commission, 1985).

Government of India, *Eighth Five Year Plan,* (New Delhi, Planning Commission, 1992).

Government of India, *Ninth Five Year Plan,* (New Delhi, Planning Commission, 1997).

Government of India, *Tenth Five Year Plan,* (New Delhi, Planning Commission, 2002).

Government of Maharashtra, *Performance Budget* – Public Health Department, 2002-2003.

Health Status, 2002 (Public Health Department, Government of Maharashtra).

National Family Health Survey, 1998-99, (Mumbai International Institute of Population Sciences).

State Health Directory, 1994, (Department of Public Health, Government of Maharashtra).

United Nations, *"Program of Action – International Conference on Population and Development"*, (Cairo, 1994).

World Health Organization, Regional Office, South East Asia, *Women of South East Asia—A Health profile,* (New Delhi; 2000).

World Health Organization, *A Decade of Health Development in South-East Asia-1968-77,* (Regional Office, South East Asia, New Delhi, 1978).

Secondary Sources

Books

Anurudh Jain, *Do Population Policies Matter? – Fertility and Politics in Egypt, India, Kenya and Mexico.* (New York, Population council, 1998).

Anthony Measham and Richard Heaver, *Supplement to India's Family Welfare Program, Moving to Reproductive and Child Health Approach* (Washington, The World Bank, 1996).

Avni Amin and Margaret E. Bentley in their study *"The Influence of Gender on Rural Women's Illness and Health-seeking Strategies for Gynaecological Symptoms"* (New Delhi, Visiaar Publication, 1996).

Danida, *Evaluation of Danish Bilateral Assistance to Health 1988-1997, Poverty and Crosscutting issues,* (New Delhi, 1998).

Dileep Malvankar, Rani Bang, Abhay Bang, *Quality Reproductive Health Services in Rural India,* (India International Council on Management of population programs, 1998).

Health Watch Trust, *Community Need-based Reproductive and Child Health in India: Progress and constraints,* (New Delhi, 1999).

Janet Smith, Rob Ritzenthaler, Elizabeth Mumford, *Policy Lessons Learned in Finance and private sector participation,* Washington DC, USA. The Futures Group International, 1998.

Karen Hardee, Kokila Agarwal, Nancy Luke, Ellen Wilson, Margaret Pendzich, Marguerite Farrel, Harry Cross, *Post Cairo Reproductive Health Policies and Programs – a comparative Study of Eight Countries,* (Washington DC, USAID, 1998).

Kelley Lee, Louisiana Lush, Gill Walt and John Cleland, *Family Planning Policies and Programs in Eight Low-income Countries: A Comparative Policy,* London School of Hygiene and Tropical Medicine, University of London, 2000.

K. Srinivasan, *Regulating Reproduction in India's Population – Efforts, Results and Recommendations.* (New Delhi, Sage Publications, 1995).

Khan, M. E. and George Cernada (eds.) *Spacing as an Alternative Strategy: India's Family Welfare Program* (New Delhi: B.R. Publishing Corporation, 1996).

Margaret Catley Carlson, from Cairo to Kayoro – *Bringing Reproductive Health to a Village in Ghana,* (New York, The Population Council, 1999).

Nafis Sadik, *The State of World Population,* New York, USA, UNFPA 1999.

Nalini Paranjape, Impact of Various Schemes Related to Elementary Education: *A Comparative Study of Girls Literacy in Maharashtra and Madhya Pradesh,* (Project sponsored by the Planning Commission, Government of India, 2000).

Phyllis Tilson Piotrow, D. Lawrence Kincaid, Jose G. Rimon II and Ward Rinehart, Health Communication – *Lessons from Family Planning and Reproductive Health,* (John Hopkins School of Public Health, Praeger Publishers, 1997).

Phyllis Tilson Piotrow, Jose G. Rimon II, 'Asia's Population and Family Planning Programs: Leaders in Strategic Communication' *Asia-Pacific Population Journal.*

Population Communications International and Ohio University, '*A Community Case Study of the Effects of a Radio Soap Opera on Gender Equality, Family Size and Individual/Collective Efficacy in India,*' (Ohio University, USA, 2002).

Population communications International, *'Humraahi': An Entertainment-Education Television Soap Opera to Promote Gender Equality in Marriage, Education, Socialization and Family Life in India,* (New York, 2002).

Pravesh Sharma, "IEC inputs for project implementation – Some Lessons from Chhattisgarh", *WEP-IFAD,* India, 2002.

Ravi Duggal, *Health Sector Financing in Context of Women's Health,* (New Delhi, ISST, 1995).

R.S. Ganpathy, S. R. Ganesh, Rushikesh Maru, Samual Paul, Ram Mohan Rao, *Public Policy and Policy Analysis in India,* (New Delhi, Sage Publications, 1985).

Sanjeevani Mulay, Asha Ram and R. Nagrajan, *Reproductive and Child Health in Nasik District: a baseline survey,* (Pune, Gokhale Institute of Politics and Economics, 1999).

Saroj Pachauri, *Implementing a Reproductive Health in India: The Beginning,* (New Delhi).

Saumya Panda, *Evolution of India's Health Policy 1947-2001 An Appraisal,* (Indian Academy of Social Sciences, Allahabad, 2002).

Shephard Forman and Romita Ghosh, *Promoting Reproductive Health – Investing in Health for Development,* (London, Lynne Rienner Publishers, 2000).

Subhash Kashyap, *National Policy Studies,* (The Lok Sabha Secretariat, New Delhi, Tata Mcgraw-Hill Publishing Company Limited, 1990).

World Bank/CINI (Child in Need Institute), *Study of Initiatives for Increasing Community Involvement in Karnataka and Tamilnadu,* (New Delhi, 1998).

Articles

Bang R.A., A.T. Bang et al. 'High Prevalence of Gynecological Diseases in Rural Indian Women'. *Lancet* 1 (8629): 85-88, 1989.

Bansal R., *'Interns as Health Educators'* World Health Forum, 1995.

C. Alison McIntosh, Jason L. Finkle, 'The Cairo Conference on Population and Development: A new Paradigm?', *Population and Development Review,* Vol. 21, No. 2, June 1995.

George A. and Nandraj S., "State of Health Care in Maharashtra—A Comparative Analysis", *Economic and Political Weekly,* 1993.

Health Watch Trust, *The community needs based RCH in India: Progress and Constraints,* Jaipur, 1999.

Institute of Health Management, *District IEC Planning for RCH, Report 1,* (Aurangabad, Maharashtra, 1998).

Khale M. and Dayalchand A., Alternative approaches to MCH services, *Indian Pediatrics* (Aurangabad, Maharashtra, 1991).

Kulkarni S. and Parasuraman S. *'Status of Maternal and Child Health in Maharashtra'* paper presented in Workshop on Child Health and Family Planning Policy Issues in Maharashtra, 1997.

M.K. Hassan, M. Jayaswal and P. Hassan, 'Abstract Reproductive Health Awareness in Rural Tribal Female Adolescents' Research Study, (Ranchi University, 2001).

Peter Mayer, 'Data and Perspectives, India's Falling Sex Ratios', *Population and Development Review,* Vol. 25, No. 2, June 99.

Prakasamma M., "Implementing the RCH Program: Challenges Before Nurses", *Indian Journal of Nursing & Midwifery,* 1998.

Qadeer I., "Reproductive Health: A Public Health Perspective", *Economic and Political Weekly,* 1998.

Ramchandran V. and Visaria L. 'Emerging Issues in Reproductive Health', *Economic and Political Weekly,* 1997.

Rao K. S. Health care services in tribal areas of Andhra Pradesh: A public policy perspective, *Economic and Political Weekly,* 1998.

Ravi Duggal, "India's Family Welfare Program in the Context of a Reproductive and Child Approach—A Critique and a Viewpoint", *MFC Bulletin, No. 234-235,* Mumbai, Sept.-Oct. 1996.

Ravi Duggal, *"Population and Family Planning Policy: A Critique and a Perspective"* Paper Presented at International Conference on Population and Development, Cairo, September 1994. (Mumbai – CEHAT – 1994).

Robert D. Retherford and Vinod Mishra, 'Media Exposure Increases Contraceptive Use' *National Family Health Survey,* (Bulletin No. 7, 1997).

R. S. Ganapathy, *On Methodologies for Policy Analysis, Indian Institute of Management,* (Ahmedabad, W.P. No. 481, October 1983).

Sanjeevani Mulay, 'Demographic Transition in Maharashtra, 1980-1993', *Economic and Political Weekly,* 34 (42 & 43) 3063-3074, 1999.

Saroj Pachauri, *Defining a Reproductive Health Package for India: A Proposed Framework, South and East Asia*—Regional Working Papers, (New Delhi, The Population Council, 1995).

Saroj Pachauri, "Relationship Between AIDS and Family Planning Programs: A Rationale for Developing Integrated Reproductive Health Services', *Health Transition Review,* 1994.

Shanti Conly, 'The Missing Billions', *People and the Planet*—Vol. 6 No. 1.

Shireen Jeejibhoy, 'Reproductive Health Information in India – What are the Gaps? *Economic and Political Weekly,* 34 (42-43) 3075-3080, 1999.

Shireen Jeejibhoy, 'Addressing Women's Reproductive Health Needs: Priorities for the Family Welfare Program', *Economic and Political Weekly,* 1997.

Shireen Jeejibhoy, *Women's Education, Autonomy and Reproductive Behaviour: Experience from Developing Countries,* (Oxford, Clarendon Press 1995).

Interviews

Interviews with Health Functionaries from the Maharashtra State Public Health Department.

Newspapers

The Times of India (Mumbai).

The Indian Express (Mumbai).

Lokmat (Amaravati).

Dainik Deshonnati (Amaravati).

Index

J

K

L

M

N

U

W

Y

Z

❑❑❑